Best Practices in Child and Behavioral Health Care

CW01020695

Series Editor

Fred R. Volkmar
Yale University
New Haven, CT, USA

Best Practices in Child and Adolescent Behavioral Health Care series explores a range of topics relevant to primary care providers in managing a broad range of child and adolescent mental health problems. These include specific disorders, such as anxiety; relevant topics in related disciplines, including psychological assessment, communication assessment, and disorders; and such general topics as management of psychiatric emergencies. The series aims to provide primary care providers with leading-edge information that enables best-care management of behavioral health issues in children and adolescents. The volumes published in this series provide concise summaries of the current research base (i.e., what is known), best approaches to diagnosis and assessment, and leading evidence-based management and treatment strategies. The series also provides information and analysis that primary care providers need to understand how to interpret and implement best treatment practices and enable them to interpret and implement recommendations from specialists for children and effectively monitor interventions.

More information about this series at http://www.springer.com/series/15955

Nancy E. Moss • Lauren Moss-Racusin

Practical Guide to Child and Adolescent Psychological Testing

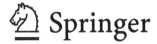 Springer

Nancy E. Moss
Yale University
New Haven, CT, USA

Lauren Moss-Racusin
Yale University
New Haven, CT, USA

ISSN 2523-7128   ISSN 2523-7136   (electronic)
Best Practices in Child and Adolescent Behavioral Health Care
ISBN 978-3-030-73517-3   ISBN 978-3-030-73515-9   (eBook)
https://doi.org/10.1007/978-3-030-73515-9

This Springer imprint is published by the registered company Springer Nature Switzerland AG
The registered company address is: Gewerbestrasse 11, 6330 Cham, Switzerland

For Gary/Dad

Acknowledgments

The authors would like to thank Drs. Lisa Wiesner, Ronald Angoff, and Cynthia Mann for their helpful suggestions. As pediatricians, their perspective on the accessibility of psychological testing was extremely valuable.

The authors would also like to thank Dr. Laurie Cardona-Wolenski for her early contributions to formulations of social-emotional test data.

Dr. Moss built her initial knowledge of psychological testing largely with the guidance of Drs. Margaret Steward and Thomas Morrison, at the University of California, Davis. Their teaching and modeling were unparalleled. Dr. Moss is particularly grateful for the mentorship of Dr. Sara Sparrow at the Yale Child Study Center. Dr. Sparrow was a towering figure in the field of psychological assessment with children and adolescents. Her wisdom underlies everything of value in this book.

Finally, the authors are grateful to the many children, adolescents, families, caregivers, and clinical colleagues who, in calling upon us to complete or interpret psychological testing, have continued to help us refine our psychological assessment skills and advance our knowledge.

About the Book

Healthcare providers have a growing role in helping parents, caregivers, children, and teens to both understand their ongoing developmental and mental health problems and to obtain needed services and support. Tackling such problems and concerns is a complex task. Psychological test data can provide much needed assistance to healthcare providers as they work to meet this challenge. Yet, because the use of psychological assessment is rarely addressed in traditional healthcare training, many healthcare providers are unfamiliar with how and when to refer patients for psychological assessment. The providers are often equally unprepared to understand and interpret psychological test results.

This book addresses this gap. It reviews the origins of psychological testing, as well as the referral process, thereby helping providers to understand the kinds of questions that can be readily addressed through testing. The book also helps providers be more specific in their referral questions to maximize the utility of the testing. The overall process of psychological assessment is discussed in detail to give providers an understanding of how assessments are done. The formal and observational data that derive from the testing, along with ways in which these data can expand an understanding of an individual's needs, are explained.

Subsequent chapters address specific domains of psychological assessment: intelligence; speech and language; visual-motor coordination; memory; attention, concentration, and executive functioning; academic achievement; behavior; adaptive functioning; social-emotional functioning; and developmental status. These sections review what these domains are, the importance of assessing them, and the most commonly encountered psychological assessment instruments for them.

Primary care providers often comment that it is challenging to know specifically what can be done to meet particular patient psychological needs, as well as the approaches that mental health practitioners, educators, caregivers, and patients could use to ameliorate identified problems. To address this challenge, in each domain's chapter, common patterns of difficulty experienced by children and adolescents are outlined, along with a summary of useful intervention approaches across a range of settings, based on assessment results. This information can aid primary care providers in their efforts to evaluate and fine-tune services offered to their patients. It is important to note that there is considerable overlap between the areas of difficulty discussed. Likewise, interventions that are outlined may be appropriate for more than one area of difficulty. These commonalities among difficulties and interventions reflect the comorbidity among disorders in child and adolescent mental health.

To facilitate critical reading and comprehension of a psychological assessment report, a fictionalized example is included at the end of this book. The purpose of this report is to pull together and demonstrate the assessment processes and components discussed throughout this book. Each section of the report is followed by in depth annotations so that the reader can see both a typical psychological assessment report along with guiding explanations. The report is written as the outcome of an independent educational evaluation (defined and explained later in this book). This type of assessment was selected, because primary care providers are likely to be involved with educators in the holistic care of school-aged youngsters and thus can benefit from a thorough orientation to this type of report. The identifying information and all other content in the report example are not representative of real individuals, for the sake of privacy and confidentiality. Any similarities to real people are coincidental.

Finally, it is important to emphasize a key foundational aspect of the material contained in this book. This book's discussion of psychological assessment is consistent with, and based upon, both contemporary research findings and many decades of clinical experience and assessment with children and adolescents. The reader can thereby gain the benefit of both empirical and practical, interpersonal knowledge and expertise.

Contents

About the Authors

Nancy E. Moss, Ph.D. Trained at the University of California and Yale University, Dr. Moss has over 30 years of experience in children's psychological testing. She has always emphasized the importance of communicating assessment findings clearly across disciplines so that medical professionals, parents, and all other caregivers can make confident, appropriate use of the findings on behalf of the children and adolescents tested. A Clinical Assistant Professor at the Yale Child Study Center, Dr. Moss combines teaching of Clinical Psychology Fellows with a long-standing private practice.

Lauren Moss-Racusin, Ph.D. After earning her undergraduate degree at Boston University, Dr. Moss-Racusin worked as a research assistant at the Yale University Consultation Center. She then completed her Ph.D. in clinical psychology at the University of Connecticut, her clinical internship at the University of Illinois at Chicago Counseling Center, and her post-graduate counseling fellowship at Temple University Tuttleman Counseling Services. She is now on staff at Yale Health Mental Health and Counseling. Dr. Moss-Racusin has focused on psychological assessment throughout her clinical training and values its integration within therapeutic practice.

Introduction

Contemporary psychological testing[1] has its roots in the early twentieth century efforts to measure intelligence in a systematic manner (Gregory, 2004). These beginning efforts expanded greatly during World War II, when the United States Armed Forces needed efficient mass screening methods to assign personnel for maximum effectiveness. Throughout the remainder of the twentieth and continuing into the twenty-first centuries, psychological assessment has developed richly. There has been tremendous growth in the number of functional domains that can be examined (Gregory, 2004).

At the same time, markedly increased conceptual and statistical sophistication, along with improved cultural and socioeconomic sensitivity, have allowed for greater confidence in assessment findings (Gregory, 2004). Historically, there have been various criticisms of psychological testing. Many of these criticisms have centered on racial, ethnic, and socioeconomic bias considered inherent in prominent assessment instruments (Gould, 1996). The challenges to psychological assessment have argued, validly, against ranking whole groups of people based on their performance on less than perfect, and sometimes mal-intended, instruments.

Contemporary test instruments are well standardized (i.e., normed on representative populations), such that test findings make it possible to determine how a given individual ranks in relation to fair expectations for someone of their age and developmental level. The instruments are generally standardized on populations that mirror current census data. With such standardization, it would be reasonable to expect that the statistical properties of the final test materials take into account racial, ethnic, and cultural diversity. However, formal psychological tests do remain vulnerable to criticism regarding structural bias in favor of dominant beliefs and practices,

---

[1] It should be noted that several terms are commonly used to refer to formal appraisal of a youngster's functioning. Psychological testing, psychological assessment, and psychological evaluation can all refer to a structured, standardized examination of multidimensional strengths and weaknesses. Throughout this book, these terms are used interchangeably.

© Springer Nature Switzerland AG 2021
N. E. Moss, L. Moss-Racusin, *Practical Guide to Child and Adolescent Psychological Testing*, Best Practices in Child and Adolescent Behavioral Health Care, https://doi.org/10.1007/978-3-030-73515-9_1

and of groups with sociopolitical privileges. Preparation for formal education, scholastic opportunities, familiarity with test-taking procedures, economic support, and extent to which the youth feels accepted and comfortable in the assessment setting are just some of the variables that may have a strong impact on psychological test results.

Fortunately, as test construction has become more sophisticated over the years, the likelihood that psychological test instruments favor individuals from dominant cultural groups, and stigmatize those from more marginalized groups, has reduced (Zurcher, 1998). The authors of this book fervently oppose any hierarchical classification of whole groups of people. Rather, information offered in this book rests on the assumption that, at the individual level, psychological test data can provide a very detailed description of a single person's strengths and weaknesses and then guide appropriate, genuinely beneficial interventions. The authors also wish to emphasize that to be truly useful, when interpreting psychological test results, careful consideration must be given to the sociodemographic factors that have potential relevance to the test outcomes.

Current psychological testing should be understood as an objective and well-structured set of procedures. These procedures involve the use of assessment instruments that are shown to be both reliable (i.e., capable of generating reproducible findings) and valid (i.e., capable of producing accurate data about the identified domains of functioning). The instruments vary in format. Some involve straightforward questions and answers. Others call for manipulation of concrete materials, completion of paper-and-pencil checklists and tests, online responses, physical enactment of responses to prompts, and/or management of open-ended inquiry. While informal evaluation and therapeutic interaction also yield important information about a youth's presentation, such clinical data are often somewhat subjective and limited by the unique interaction between particular caregivers or providers and youngsters. In contrast, psychological assessment findings provide clear, verifiable information that goes beyond the boundaries of a single interaction.

Psychological testing offers a major contribution to primary care practice and to a wide array of community-based medical, mental health, and child welfare organizations. Providers in such settings are continually required to make complicated, critically important decisions about patient or client welfare. Often, these decisions have to be made in the midst of multiple other professional demands and with painfully little time. Such a decision-making process is often very stressful. Appropriate use of psychological assessment can relieve some of this stress. Results from a psychological assessment can ground direct practice in a solid understanding of an individual child or adolescent. A youth's behavior is often much more understandable when seen in the context of their comprehensive portrait, as contained in the test results.

Furthermore, assessment findings can help guide interventions. With ongoing reference to the test findings, providers can be more confident that their intervention-planning and decision-making are most consistent with a youth's identified strengths, problem areas, and needs. In addition, findings from assessments and reassessments can help providers track progress and development, to ensure that interventions proceed in the most productive direction. Collaboration with the examiner who carries out the psychological assessment also provides primary care providers with another professional colleague whose consultation can be supportive and informative.

References

Gould, S. J. (1996). *The mismeasure of man*. W. W. Norton and Company.

Gregory, R. J. (2004). *Psychological testing: History, principles, and applications*. Allyn & Bacon.

Zurcher, R. (1998). Issues and trends in culture-fair assessment. *Intervention in School and Clinic, 34*(2). https://doi.org/10.1177/105345129803400206

Types of Psychological Assessments

When providers, educators, and/or parents or caregivers are making a psychological testing referral for children and adolescents, there is often question about whether to request a clinical psychological assessment, a neuropsychological assessment, or school psychoeducational testing. There is considerable overlap among these three types of evaluation, since all testing of young individuals must focus on documenting developmental status and progress. Yet, there are some important differences among these types in regard to their primary focus and to the nature of their recommendations. Each type has both advantages and drawbacks. Guidance is provided below about making suitable referral choices.

Clinical Psychological Assessment

A clinical psychological assessment is most often conducted by a doctoral level clinical psychologist located in a medical or mental health organization or in a private practice setting. Such an assessment may focus on a wide range of developmental domains. This range typically includes intelligence, related cognitive capacities, speech and language, visual-motor coordination, attention and concentration, executive functioning, behavioral functioning, social-emotional condition, and developmental status. Specific domains to be examined are designated on a case-by-case basis depending on particular referral questions. Relevant diagnostic, educational, and treatment recommendations are generated in relation to the most salient findings.

The advantages of obtaining a clinical psychological assessment pertain to the generally high level of examiner expertise, privacy afforded by the setting in which this type of assessment is commonly carried out, comprehensive nature of the testing, as well as both the breadth and depth of findings regarding the youth's personality functioning and social-emotional strengths and problem areas. The drawbacks of

© Springer Nature Switzerland AG 2021
N. E. Moss, L. Moss-Racusin, *Practical Guide to Child and Adolescent Psychological Testing*, Best Practices in Child and Adolescent Behavioral Health Care, https://doi.org/10.1007/978-3-030-73515-9_2

a comprehensive clinical psychological assessment involve first a considerable financial expenditure. Second, for cases in which school performance is an issue, having assessment done by a private practitioner then requires delicate consultations in order to incorporate the findings into the educational programming. In the great majority of situations, though, the consultation can be carried out successfully.

Neuropsychological Assessment

In requesting a neuropsychological assessment for a youngster, the hope is generally to learn a great deal about their fundamental developmental capacities and rankings. There are clear characteristics of a neuropsychological assessment. As with the clinical psychological assessment, this type of assessment is most often carried out by a doctoral level psychologist, with specialized training in neuropsychology. Also as with clinical psychological assessments, the practitioner is located either in an organizational or private practice setting. The neuropsychological assessment is organized differently than the clinical psychological assessment, though. Whereas clinical psychological testing focuses on individual functioning in a range of developmental domains, neuropsychological assessment focuses on particular brain functions (e.g., memory, visual processing, etc.), and their relationships to observable behavior. Most of the time, neuropsychological assessment generates comprehensive recommendations designed to guide treatment of, and accommodation to, the deficits identified in the testing.

Clinical psychological assessment advantages noted above, involving examiner level of training and expertise, privacy, and the comprehensive nature of the testing, are also assets of a neuropsychological assessment. The prime advantage of the latter, though, is that it yields invaluable information in cases of suspected brain abnormality and/or injury. For example, in cases involving concussions (i.e., a mild form of traumatic brain injury usually incurred during vigorous physical activity), neuropsychological assessment can help explain resultant persistent physical symptoms, as well as functional impacts across diverse cognitive and behavioral skills. Used in combination with contemporary brain imaging, neuropsychological assessment can also enhance treatment of significant neurological illness or damage.

Neuropsychological assessment also has drawbacks. As with clinical psychological assessment, neuropsychological testing is generally quite expensive. Careful consultation is also required for integration of neuropsychological test findings into educational program-planning. In addition, neuropsychologists have relatively little training in the evaluation of social-emotional functioning. As a result, the neuropsychological assessment findings often have much less to offer to assist with addressing social-emotional concerns.

School Psychoeducational Testing

The aim of school psychoeducational testing is to better understand students' struggles and to optimize their educational progress. Both public and private school students are eligible for school psychoeducational testing, since public school systems are legally mandated to meet the designated special needs of students attending all schools located in the systems' districts. The testing is administered by school psychologists, who are employees of the school district, and most of whom are trained at the Master's level. However, some school psychologists hold doctoral degrees, as well. In contrast to clinical psychological and neuropsychological assessments, school psychoeducational assessments are usually more limited in scope, focusing closely on determining the sources of observed academic struggles.

School psychologists are able to capitalize on their specialized knowledge of educational demands, and on their extensive familiarity with academic functioning, in order to interpret test results in a useful manner. There is, however, quite a bit of variability regarding generation of recommendations based on school psychoeducational testing. This variability relates to the fact that the school psychologist always functions as a member of a multidisciplinary educational team. The team is typically composed of special education administrators, regular and special education teachers, speech-language specialists, occupational therapists, physical therapists and behavior analysts, along with the psychologist. School districts differ in their approach to integrating team members' contributions. In some districts, each team member operates somewhat independently. In such a district, the school psychologist generates a report that concludes with a set of recommendations related specifically to the psychoeducational test data obtained. In other districts, though, administrators prefer to have the educational team, as a whole, generate a set of recommendations based on an integration of all the team members' findings. These recommendations are then included in records documenting the broad special education process (i.e., Individualized Educational Plans). In such a district, the school psychologist's recommendations are meant to be reflected in the multidisciplinary formulation of a student's psychoeducational needs and relevant services.

There are two main advantages to obtaining a school psychoeducational assessment. The first involves finances: this type of assessment is carried out at no cost to parents or caregivers. The second advantage involves the school district's greater willingness to use the data gathered. Since the assessment is administered by a representative of the district, the district often has more trust in the data's accuracy, such that there is minimal need for delicate consultations.

As with the other types of assessments, there are also drawbacks to relying on school psychoeducational testing. Parents and caregivers have far less capacity to maintain privacy about the assessment process and its results. Additionally, given the typical level of school psychologist training, as well as the typical scope of school psychoeducational assessments, they are much less comprehensive than other types of testing. Finally, district financial and administrative concerns may impact the district's decisions about how the assessment is conducted and how the results are interpreted. To illustrate, other than diagnoses of Intellectual Disability and Specific Learning Disorder, school districts generally refrain from offering diagnostic formulations. When additional symptomatology appears present, a school district will typically only go as far as suggesting family consultation with private professionals. At times, the impacts of these drawbacks can be lessened by cooperative efforts between the school psychologist and a private clinical psychologist or neuropsychologist.

Independent Educational Evaluation

In most situations, families, other caregivers, and educators can come together to plan acceptably for administration and interpretation of appropriate psychological assessments, followed by cooperative design of a useful educational program. However, in some situations, the adults involved with a particular youngster cannot come to agreement. Sometimes, there is a worry that the district personnel cannot adequately and accurately assess a youngster's difficulties. At other times, there is frank disagreement about the nature of the youngster's problems. In still other situations, educators and caregivers have widely different levels of concern about a child or adolescent's functioning. It may also be the case that those involved with a youngster have contradictory interpretations of data already generated.

In such cases, the district and caregivers may decide together to pursue an independent educational evaluation, paid for by the school district. If this decision is made, the school personnel and the caregivers together choose an appropriate examiner and determine the information they are hoping to obtain. Everyone involved then agrees to accept the results of the evaluation. An independent educational evaluation is most often administered by a private, doctoral level psychologist. The scope of the evaluation is generally quite comprehensive, and a wide range of pertinent recommendations is offered based on the assessment findings.

Court-Ordered Assessments

Although this area is not a focus of this book, it is important to note that children and adolescents involved with the legal system sometimes require psychological assessment. Testing is usually required when the Court has questions about a youngster's condition relevant to the issues up for judgment. In some instances, psychological testing can be used to examine the impact of specified events or situations on a youngster. For example, in cases of alleged abuse, results of psychological assessment can document the youngster's traumatic experience and its consequences. Youngsters caught in caregiver custody and visitation disputes can also benefit from psychological testing. In such situations, the psychological test data can highlight the youngster's critical areas of need and clarify their views of their relationships with their caregivers. In other instances, when the youngster is the individual accused of illegal action, questions often arise regarding true responsibility for behaviors that have been carried out. Psychological test findings can help explain the sources of the child or adolescent's behavior and assist in determining their mental capacity to understand their actions.

When the Court determines that psychological test information is needed, it orders a psychological assessment. The specific nature of the assessment depends on the concrete issues confronting particular children and adolescents. It is imperative that everyone connected to the case understands that all findings will be shared with the Court. In carrying out a court-ordered assessment, a psychologist must conduct the assessment in the most suitable setting, be that a clinical office, a place more familiar and comfortable for the youngster, or jail; gather all pertinent background information; and consult with all parties involved. Furthermore, the psychologist must offer an opinion about the youngster's ability and willingness to participate in a truthful, forthright manner. The report of such an assessment includes explicit recommendations for the Court's consideration.

Referral Process

When to Refer for Psychological Assessment

There is a wide array of situations that call for psychological assessment. When primary care providers encounter one of them, a referral for psychological testing can enhance quality of care and treatment outcomes. These situations are discussed below.

Individual Child/Adolescent

In working with a child or adolescent, questions can arise regarding a large number of personal characteristics. Psychological testing is an excellent resource for explaining the sources and effects of these characteristics. More specifically, psychological assessment findings can shed light on a youngster's intelligence level, broader cognitive strengths and problem areas, language skills, visual-motor coordination, executive functioning, memory operations, general behavioral functioning, adaptive behavior, social-emotional adjustment, and developmental status. When problems are identified, the test results can document their nature and severity level. Relevant recommendations based on the findings then pinpoint specific strategies and interventions to improve the youngster's situation.

Family Issues

Often, primary care providers note aspects of family functioning and relationships that may have a negative impact on a child or adolescent. Caregiver disciplinary style, poor caregiver-child communication, extreme sibling conflict, hostility

© Springer Nature Switzerland AG 2021   11
N. E. Moss, L. Moss-Racusin, *Practical Guide to Child and Adolescent Psychological Testing*, Best Practices in Child and Adolescent Behavioral Health Care, https://doi.org/10.1007/978-3-030-73515-9_3

between caregivers, management of daily practical needs, family exposure to socioeconomic hardship, and violence are some examples of the aspects of family life that may provoke questions in the minds of providers. For the greatest accuracy in addressing child or adolescent problems, the significance of such aspects of family functioning need to be well understood. Typically, though, limitations imposed by scheduling demands and the nature of the primary care relationship prevent full exploration of these family characteristics within the framework of regular clinical contact. Individualized psychological testing can supplement primary care by detailing the particular effects of family functioning on an individual child or adolescent. Furthermore, psychological assessment findings can provide information about how a particular youth may challenge or enhance family functioning.

School Problems

In seeking service from a primary care provider, parents and caregivers commonly voice worries about both a youngster's behavior in school and their academic performance. Psychological testing can be particularly helpful in identifying the underlying sources of problematic behavior and in explaining the obstacles to better academic achievement.

In regard to problematic behavior, casual observation of unacceptable behavior often leads adults to conclude that youngsters are simply seeking attention. The drive to get attention is assumed to be so strong that youngsters are believed to prefer negative attention to an absence of attention. Indeed, many years of research findings provide ample empirical support for this belief, and in some cases, youngsters are driven to obtain any sort of attention (e.g., Mellor, 2008). However, it would be wrong to conclude that all inappropriate behavior is exclusively or primarily attention-seeking. In a large number of cases, unacceptable behavior is best understood as a manifestation of underlying, enduring diagnoses. Occasionally, the unacceptable behavior actually represents the youngster's effort to shift adult attention away from a diagnostic status that is a source of shame or embarrassment for the young person. Adult responses that target only the rule-breaking and attention-seeking aspects of undesirable behaviors risk being unduly punitive while ignoring the more fundamental and important aspects of the youngster's development. Psychological testing is an excellent tool for accurately identifying relevant diagnoses, linking them to observed behaviors, and thereby providing guidance toward appropriate interventions.

Regarding academic achievement difficulties, youngsters display poor scholastic accomplishments for a variety of reasons. These include inferior instruction, low quality curriculum materials, Learning Disorders (i.e., inability to adequately process particular types of information), intrusive psychological or emotional concerns, behavioral disruption, teacher-student incompatibility, and distressing peer relationships. Interaction with, and observation of, the student in the classroom are alone often insufficient to distinguish among these potential contributors to academic struggles. Psychological testing, however, can make these distinctions precisely, and again, guide parents, caregivers, and educators toward the most useful interventions.

Program/Resource Eligibility

Primary care providers may also encounter children and adolescents with presentations that warrant or even require certain programmatic interventions. For example, local, state, and federal resources are mandated for children and adolescents who meet designated criteria (e.g., who have diagnoses of Intellectual Disability and/or Autism Spectrum Disorder). Some youngsters require accommodations (e.g., extended time on exams or private testing locations) in order to fully display their true potential and ability, and thereby continue on a successful academic trajectory. Additionally, on occasion, youngsters may be intellectually gifted, and specialized programs exist to enhance the development of those with much greater than typical intellectual capacity. Psychological testing is one of the best ways to document a young person's eligibility for both necessary and/or desired services and accommodations.

"Intractable" Cases

Inevitably in the course of primary care service delivery, providers encounter children and adolescents who respond poorly to an array of interventions on their behalf, or who have poor compliance with treatment protocols. Providers, caregivers, and youngsters may all experience frustration in the face of limited progress or even a worsening of a youngster's situation, especially when a reasonable explanation is not readily apparent. To help avoid physical and psychological suffering, conflictual relationships, as well as premature termination of services, a referral for psychological testing can often result in identifying unknown clinical factors. A better understanding of such clinical factors can help providers, caregivers, and youth shift their efforts in a more productive direction.

Specific Referral Questions

When responding to a request for psychological testing, a psychologist who provides psychological assessment services has an impressive breadth and depth of knowledge on which to draw. The psychologist also has a wide array of test instruments from which to choose. Much of the psychologist's skill is directed at activating their most relevant knowledge and making wise choices regarding specific test instruments. To carry out these functions most efficiently and helpfully for a particular patient, the psychologist must be guided by the most precise referral questions possible. Without such guidance, the psychologist is left to assess, without specific focus or purpose, a wide array of patient strengths and problem areas. Such a far-reaching assessment is vulnerable to missing the most important aspects of a specific patient's presentation.

As discussed in the Clinical Psychological/Neuropsychological Assessment Process chapter, it is best if referral questions can be developed directly with parents or caregivers. However, there are situations in which this responsibility falls solely or primarily to primary care providers, or in which primary care providers (with legal permission) share additional questions with the psychologist. For a referring provider, a straightforward case review can usually facilitate generation of appropriate referral questions. Consistent with the clinical presentations discussed above, specification of problem areas in a patient's personal, relational, and academic functioning; outline of gaps in knowledge about the patient; identification of roadblocks in delivering primary care; and designation of pieces of information needed for treatment-planning all serve to help formulate useful referral questions.

To illustrate, a child might present in primary care as non-compliant with nutritional plans for obesity control. Psychological testing to determine "what is going on with this child" might, but also might not, hit upon the most likely explanations for the non-compliance. In contrast, a request to distinguish between the potential contributions to non-compliance of confusion about treatment due to limited intellectual capacity versus of interference from emerging psychotic symptoms would elicit much better assessment service from a psychologist.

Collegial Relationships

Just as design of precise referral questions enhances the potential usefulness of psychological assessment, so, too, does maintenance of ongoing consultative relationships. It is very helpful for primary care providers and assessing psychologists to establish close, collegial ties. The primary care providers can educate the psychologists about the nature of their medical practice and the characteristics of their patient population. In turn, the psychologists can educate their primary care colleagues about the scope of psychological testing, interpretation of commonly used tests, and design of clinical recommendations. Such mutual understanding helps to ensure that psychological testing is conducted at the right level, in the most useful way, and in the most accurate context. Ultimately, multidisciplinary collaboration with open communication and frequent interaction allows patients to benefit significantly.

Reference

Mellor, N. (2008). *Attention seeking: A complete guide for teachers* (2nd ed.). Sage Publications Inc.

Clinical Psychological/Neuropsychological Assessment Process

In this chapter, the actual process of the assessment is discussed. It is important to understand that the purpose of each step is to facilitate the comprehensive understanding of the child or adolescent, the final well-informed acceptance of the findings, and the willingness to implement the recommendations on behalf of the youngster. The assessment consists of the following steps, which are explicated below.

1. Request for Testing
2. Initial Appointment
3. School/Home Observation, as needed
4. Professional Consultation
5. Direct Assessment
6. Interpretive Meeting(s)
7. Generation and Dissemination of Written Report
8. Follow-Up Consultation, as needed
9. Reassessment, as needed

Request for Testing

The psychological assessment process begins by contacting a psychologist to request testing. It is best for this request to be conveyed directly from the parent(s) or caregiver(s) most closely involved with the child or adolescent. Rather than being a formality, the experience of communicating the request enhances the parent or caregiver's later openness to thoughtful consideration of the test findings.

There are two main goals in this initial contact. First, the psychologist must determine that they are qualified to carry out the necessary testing. For this determination to be made, a brief description of the presenting problems and broad referral

© Springer Nature Switzerland AG 2021   17
N. E. Moss, L. Moss-Racusin, *Practical Guide to Child and Adolescent Psychological Testing*, Best Practices in Child and Adolescent Behavioral Health Care, https://doi.org/10.1007/978-3-030-73515-9_4

questions needs to be presented. The psychologist assesses the goodness-of-fit between these problems and questions, on one hand, and the psychologist's qualifications, on the other hand. If the psychologist's training does not equip them to address the issues at hand, a more appropriate referral is offered. If the psychologist is able to carry out the necessary assessment well, then planning proceeds.

Once the psychologist has determined that they can offer the testing, the focus of discussion can shift to the second goal, which is to attend to practical considerations for the assessment. Office accessibility, scheduling, fees, payment options, and possible insurance coverage are all discussed. It is essential that these components of the assessment be agreed upon at this early stage. Without such agreement, there is a real risk that the assessment will be terminated prematurely or that the ultimate findings will be disregarded. Either negative outcome is detrimental to the youngster in need of assistance. Again, if this second goal cannot be achieved, the psychologist takes responsibility for referring to a colleague for services that are hopefully better aligned. Assuming, though, that both goals of the initial contact are met successfully, a first appointment can be arranged to begin the assessment.

Initial Appointment

The initial appointment is aimed at setting the foundation for the assessment. In this meeting, the discussion focuses on obtaining a full sense of the concerns that prompted the request for testing so that appropriate, specific referral questions can be developed. At the outset of the meeting, the adult(s) requesting the assessment are invited to share their primary concerns regarding the youngster. The discussion of these concerns is now more comprehensive than was possible during the initial contact described above. The psychologist listens carefully to all that the parents or caregivers have to relate. When ready, the psychologist reflects back their under standing in order to guarantee a shared purpose in undertaking the testing. Any misunderstandings should be corrected. Based on mutual grasp of the concerns, specific and concrete referral questions are identified. These questions ensure that test selection, administration, and final interpretation are appropriately individualized and relevant to the youngster.

Once the referral questions have been properly formulated, attention is then shifted to obtaining as complete a developmental history as possible. If biological parents are initiating the assessment, full developmental information is usually available. If the assessment is being supported by other caregivers, the developmental history may be less complete.

The developmental history provides a context for correct interpretation of the data at the conclusion of direct testing. To be most useful for later data interpretation, the developmental history should include a detailed description of the pregnancy, labor, and delivery, highlighting any concerning events or problematic medical test findings. Birthweight and the newborn's overall condition (as indexed by APGAR scores, if known) are noted. Infant and toddler characteristics are then discussed. Feeding methods and ease of feeding, sleeping patterns, and the capacity to be soothed when necessary are the most important characteristics to investigate.

Following consideration of these early characteristics, the youngster's achievements of early developmental milestones are then assessed. First use of pointing in order to convey information to another, first independent walking, first use of single words, first communication via phrases and sentences, and toilet training are the milestones that many parents and caregivers can recall reliably. Childcare arrangements from birth through the time of the assessment are reviewed; these arrangements include preschool attendance along with later school placements and progress. Any significant medical illnesses, as well as major accidents, are also discussed.

Medical and psychological history in the extended family is examined in order to note any conditions to which the youngster might be vulnerable. Familial experience of attention disorders, Learning Disorders, neurological diseases, cognitive impairments, speech-language disorders, eating disorders, Autism Spectrum Disorder, psychiatric diagnoses, behavior problems, alcoholism or other substance abuse, and chronic illnesses are particularly important to note. If the youngster was adopted, the psychologist inquires briefly about the circumstances that led to the adoption and gathers whatever information is known about the pregnancy, labor, and delivery, as well as the extended biological family history.

Caregivers often feel relieved if the discussion of the developmental history can conclude with a more pleasant topic. Accordingly, it is useful to ask, for example, about how the youngster's name was chosen. Caregivers are generally quite happy to relive their own decision-making process, or what they know of another's. By attending carefully to their report, the psychologist can learn important information about family values, culture, and problem-solving style. Religious convictions, a wish to honor preceding generations, fascination with literary or theatrical figures, the desire to identify a name comfortable in multiple languages, and attachments to individuals involved in labor and delivery are among the variables often cited as reasons for name choices.

At the conclusion of the initial appointment, parents and caregivers often ask about the best way to prepare their youngster for the assessment. They wonder what should be said to maximize the youngster's comfort and thereby help to elicit the highest quality performance from them. In response to this inquiry, it is best to encourage honest, forthright explanations. Usually, children and adolescents are calmed by hearing that caregivers (along with medical providers and teachers, when relevant) wish to obtain all the knowledge they need to ensure that the youth is receiving all assistance necessary. It is helpful to emphasize that the testing is aimed at making constructive recommendations rather than highlighting possible weaknesses, and that no painful physical procedures are part of the psychological assessment. The youngster can be reassured further by learning that there will be no grades or homework assigned, and that the psychologist will be supportive throughout the assessment.

Throughout this initial meeting, the psychologist is attending carefully to parent or caregiver style, tone, vocabulary, and apparent intellectual level. The psychologist then uses this information to attune to, and best engage and connect with, the caregivers for the remainder of the assessment. By relating in the manner most familiar and comfortable for the adults involved, the psychologist helps to ensure that the test findings will be well understood and accepted, and that recommendations will be implemented.

School/Home Observation

In some cases, initial discussion raises significant concern about a child or adolescent's ability to fully display their strengths and vulnerabilities in the formal assessment setting. An excessive need for sameness, a high level of generalized anxiety, fear of strangers, or markedly unusual behavior requiring familiarity with the youngster for correct interpretation are among the main sources of concern about beginning the assessment in the testing setting. It is probable that observation in a comfortable, familiar setting will provide the most accurate introduction to the typical functioning of such a youngster.

Once it is determined that an observation would be useful, the observation should occur before the psychologist and youngster begin working closely together. Observing before becoming well known to the youngster allows for gathering the most realistic information. Whether in the home or school environment, the psychologist watches quietly from the background. Note-taking is done as unobtrusively as possible. If the child or adolescent or a peer approaches, the psychologist responds pleasantly but minimally.

The observation focuses on several behavioral dimensions. These include the youngster's capacity to participate appropriately in the activities at hand, interpersonal interaction style, communication skills, behavioral self-control, need for assistance, as well as willingness and ability to use assistance. The psychologist notes both the ways in which others in the environment have come to relate to the youngster, as well as the extent to which the environment has been modified to accommodate the youngster. To help guarantee reasonable interpretation, the observation concludes with a brief conversation with a caregiver or teacher to determine how typical the observed behavior was. Considerations about whether the observed behavior was consistent with overall functioning, dramatically worse in response to the pressure of the psychologist's presence or some other factor, or significantly better due to extreme effort to impress the psychologist are all incorporated into an initial understanding of the youngster.

Professional Consultation

In some cases, a child or adolescent is already involved with other professionals. These professionals most typically include pediatricians, related medical care providers, subspecialty physicians, nurses, psychotherapists, occupational therapists, physical therapists, speech-language specialists, and teachers. Often, these individuals possess invaluable information about the youngster's history, current struggles, and family functioning. Obtaining this information provides critical assistance in focusing the assessment. With permission from caregivers, and from older adolescents themselves, the psychologist can carefully consult with all relevant professionals and incorporate their information into the overall assessment.

Direct Assessment

Once the foundation has been laid for the assessment, as described above, the direct assessment with the youngster can begin. Four to six sessions are typically required for a comprehensive assessment. These sessions are scheduled at intervals, times of day, and durations best suited to the youth being tested. To safeguard the integrity of the test results, the psychologist adheres to standardized testing procedures. Within the standard framework, though, the psychologist does everything possible to help the youngster feel comfortable and supported. For example, in some cases, in order to maximize test performance, formal testing is alternated with play periods. The play periods provide relief to youngsters and may also aid in diagnostic formulation.

In the assessment setting, the psychologist and youth sit at a clear work table in a quiet, private environment. Generally, the assessment begins with the psychologist going back over the preparatory information provided to the youngster earlier by a parent or caregiver. Testing then starts with what would likely be a relatively easy task for a particular child or adolescent. This initial low level of difficulty allows the youth to settle more comfortably into the assessment. The assessment then addresses each developmental domain relevant to the referral questions. As discussed in later chapters, these domains include intellectual functioning, speech-language skills, visual-motor coordination, memory, attentional and executive functioning, academic achievement, behavioral characteristics, social-emotional status, and developmental capacity. The psychologist carefully monitors the youth's assessment performance and makes any necessary adjustments in test instrument choice.

Occasionally, a parent or caregiver needs to remain in the room where the testing is being conducted. There are four main reasons why the presence of the parent or caregiver may be necessary. First, the youngster might be too anxious to separate. Extreme anxiety is seen most often in very young children or in older children or adolescents who carry diagnoses that have an anxiety component. In such cases, it is most helpful for all adults involved to have a matter-of-fact attitude. The youngster is encouraged to engage independently in the testing, but when needed, the reassuring presence of a known, trusted adult can be allowed in a calm, supportive manner. Often, with this type of support at the outset of an assessment, the youngster becomes able to separate easily in later test sessions.

Second, there are cases in which it is the parents or caregivers who are too anxious to separate. These parents or caregivers find it difficult to trust another adult (i.e., the psychologist) to behave safely and appropriately with their youngster. For such individuals, it is best to allow them to remain in the assessment setting to monitor the proceedings. Opposing their wishes would only increase their distrust and could potentially then deprive the youngster of much needed assessment. As with anxious youngsters, when allowed to be present for the initial test sessions, many caregivers become sufficiently comfortable to allow the remainder of the assessment to continue without their supervision.

The need for interpretation of a youngster's communication and related behaviors is the third reason for a parent or caregiver to remain in the testing room. For some children and adolescents, level of functioning and diagnostic presentations involve unclear verbalizations and unusual behaviors. The psychologist might lack sufficient familiarity with the youngster to accurately understand what is being communicated or displayed, leading to psychologist errors in judgment and interpretation. Such errors would distort the final test findings. While it is possible that the communication and/or behavior is truly too disorganized to comprehend, many times those who know the child or adolescent best do understand readily and fully. Learning from their understanding allows the psychologist to most accurately interpret the youngster's response to test instruments.

Finally, the fourth reason for a parent or caregiver to remain in the assessment setting has to do with behavior management. There are youngsters whose behavioral and emotional problems raise concern about potentially dangerous acting out in the assessment setting. For such youngsters, the presence of a familiar adult can often have a calming effect, thereby avoiding acting out behaviors. On the rare occasions when acting out still occurs, the familiar adult and the psychologist designing individualized behavior management strategies can usually guarantee everyone's safety.

Regardless of the reason for the parent or caregiver's presence, it is essential that they refrain from providing answers to test items and/or from rephrasing test items to enhance a youngster's test performance. Refraining from "helping" the youngster is often painfully difficult for the parent or caregiver. It is very uncomfortable for a caring adult to watch a youngster struggle or even fail during testing. The psychologist can provide support for the caregiver to minimize their discomfort.

Interpretive Meetings

When direct assessment is complete, a psychologist needs some time to score instruments and interpret findings. Once this work is finished, a meeting can be arranged to provide feedback to parents or caregivers. This interpretive meeting is the culmination of all of the assessment efforts; it is the setting in which the essential information originally requested is conveyed, and in which guidance is offered about how best to help the youth. Such a meeting typically lasts approximately one hour. Beyond this duration, fatigue compromises both professional performance and parent or caregiver comprehension. If further discussion is necessary after the hour has passed, another meeting can be scheduled.

It is common for parents or caregivers to be quite anxious at interpretive meetings. The information to be discussed is intimately important, and thus anxiety is fully understandable. To help relieve anxiety (as noted above in relation to the initial appointment), the psychologist can adjust their demeanor, vocabulary, and communication style to match those of the caregivers as closely as possible. This adjustment helps the caregivers to comprehend the information being shared, to feel well understood, and to be comfortable speaking.

To provide additional anxiety relief, the psychologist should offer the caregivers three main options for how to structure the interpretive meeting. The first is for the psychologist to discuss, at length, the process and outcome of the assessment, noting the youth's behavior and level of cooperation, listing the domains assessed and the instruments used, outlining the important results, offering in-depth interpretations, making recommendations, and then answering questions. This approach is the most thorough and organized. Some parents or caregivers feel burdened by so much information, though, and can instead choose between the remaining two options. The caregivers can name their most pressing current concerns, requesting that the psychologist address these concerns first. Additional feedback can then be provided, as relevant. Responding to the most pressing worry at the beginning of the discussion often allows the parents or caregivers to relax a bit, and thus enhances their ability to engage more easily in the overall interpretive meeting. The final option is to forego any detailed presentation of scores and concrete test performance in favor of the psychologist engaging immediately in a blunt discussion of the essential core of the findings and the relevant recommendations.

In whatever fashion the caregivers select, the psychologist should fulfill their responsibility to talk frankly about the test results and their meaning, significance, and implications. Doing so often involves sensitive conversations that demand of the psychologist tact and empathy for the impact of the findings being conveyed. Caregivers can and should expect a clear conversation with assessment findings delivered honestly and respectfully. Furthermore, caregivers also have a right to expect support and compassion regarding any disturbing assessment results. The psychologist should inquire directly about whether or not the caregivers believe that their initial referral questions were answered.

The interpretive meeting concludes with discussion of concrete recommendations intended to guide parents and caregivers toward explicit changes to improve the lives of their youngster and of themselves. Caregivers vary greatly in their wishes about acting on the psychologist's recommendations. Sometimes, the interpretive meeting ends with a clear plan of action for implementing all of the recommendations. In other cases, caregivers choose to take time to absorb the findings and then decide how to proceed. For some people, the data are sufficiently complex that the interpretive is spread over more than one meeting. There are also times when caregivers choose not to follow the psychologist's recommendations. Good-faith disagreement about the youth's best interest, conflicting advice from other professionals, personal caregiver discomfort, and/or defensive refusal to accept the data and recommendations are all possible reasons for bypassing the psychologist's recommendations. It is most important that, no matter the direction they choose, caregivers leave the interpretive meeting(s) feeling that their original questions were addressed and that they received understandable, useful information.

When children and adolescents are both interested in and capable of understanding test findings, the results can be shared with them in a briefer, follow-up meeting. Unless an older adolescent insists on a private meeting, parents or caregivers should be present in order to ensure that everyone has received the same information. Presentation of the findings to children and adolescents should emphasize praise and support for their test participation. Youth are provided with a condensed version of the overall assessment findings (i.e., the three or four main elements). These core findings are discussed truthfully and supportively. Even the most troubling findings can be phrased in a hopeful way that highlights the youth's strengths. Recommendations are then reviewed using concepts and vocabulary understandable to the youth. Questions and reactions from the youngster are explored. It is often most productive to ask the child or adolescent whether any of the findings surprised them. Many times, their answers to this question provide an opening into their most significant thoughts and fears about themselves. Overall, a well-informed child or adolescent is usually best equipped to accept, and cooperate with, interventions on their behalf.

Generation and Dissemination of the Written Report

When all phases of the assessment are done, the psychologist and caregivers discuss and come to agreement about whether a written report would be useful. In almost all cases, it is best to have a comprehensive written report that summarizes all aspects of the assessment and includes the recommendations. In a small minority of cases, though, caregivers elect to forgo receiving a written report. A decision against obtaining a written report usually reflects caregivers' budgetary concerns, wishes for extreme privacy, or intentions to withhold assessment information from individuals or organizations believed to be less than fully supportive of a child or adolescent.

In some instances, the psychologist and caregivers may decide that multiple versions of a report would be desirable. This is most often the case when the full clinical report contains a great deal of intensely personal background or diagnostic information. Caregivers and the youth themselves may prefer to share this type of information only with the healthcare professionals who most need to understand it. In such cases, an abridged version of the test report can be written to share with educators and/or others. The abridged version still contains all information necessary to appropriately guide academic and other required interventions. Overall, when requested to do so, the psychologist has the responsibility to write a test report and share it with everyone designated by the caregivers.

It is important to note here that it is extremely uncomfortable for almost every individual to read their own test report. Clinical written narrative about oneself is simply hard to bear. This discomfort is particularly acute for children and adolescents. In the interests of being protective, although youngsters should be informed about their test results, it is recommended that reading the actual report be postponed until they are older.

It is critically important to put the psychological test report to long and active use. All too often, psychological test reports are filed away without really informing ongoing interaction and work with a child or adolescent. Rather than shelving the report, caregivers, all providers involved, and the youth themselves (when old and capable enough) should use the report as a guide in psychoeducational program-planning and mental health interventions. When trying to determine the significance of a specific behavior, or when facing tough educational and clinical decisions (e.g., a possible course of treatment, the utility of medication, etc.), caregivers and professionals alike should refer back to the test report for guidance.

Follow-Up Consultation

There are cases in which the assessment findings call for input from other professionals. For example, a particular pattern of Intelligence Quotient score changes could require a neurologist to rule out the presence of a lesion in the brain. The utility of such follow-up consultation is generally outlined in the recommendations section of a psychological assessment report, or discussed as a recommendation if no report is generated. In such cases, the psychologist and the parents or caregivers might agree to pursue additional professional consultation to make sure that all of the implications of the assessment results are understood and attended to fully. The consultant uses the information from the psychological assessment to inform their consultation and to guide further recommendations.

Reassessment

Many of the questions addressed by psychological assessment of children and adolescents relate to developmental processes that unfold over a period of years. Level of intelligence, Learning Disorders, and serious mental illness are all good examples of domains that can be determined and diagnosed with greater certainty after following a youngster's course of development over time. When reassessment is included as a recommendation generated by psychological testing, it is typically with the goals of clarifying uncertain assessment findings and/or of tracking an unfolding developmental process, and with the ultimate aim of providing accurate diagnoses and appropriate guidance for interventions. In addition, qualifications for participation in some programs, whether remedial or enrichment, require up-to-date assessment data. Therefore, psychological reassessments are often necessary.

Reassessments are conducted just as initial assessments are, but they focus somewhat more closely on the specific issues that are being tracked. For reassessment to yield valid and reliable results, waiting at least one to one-and-a-half years between administrations of the same test instrument or of the same form of a test instrument is usually essential. The manuals of each test contain specific guidance on intervals. If an instrument or form is repeated prematurely, it is impossible to distinguish between true change in a youngster and evidence of their familiarity with the measure.

An exception to this timeline is in reassessment of adaptive behavior, which may be meaningfully carried out with the same instruments much more frequently than reassessment of other domains of functioning. The reason is that adaptive skills can genuinely change more rapidly than other capacities and skills. To illustrate, the Vineland Adaptive Behavior Scales (Sparrow et al., 2016) contain items pertaining to a child's skill at tying shoelaces. Upon first assessment, a child may not have this skill, but re-administration after only two weeks may validly reflect newfound independence on this developmental dimension.

Of note, if there are genuine questions about the validity of an assessment (e.g., some element of the testing setting precluded a youngster's realistic performance), then it may be impractical or distressing to wait more than a year to resolve the questions. Reassessment may be carried out sooner, as long as alternate test instruments, or alternate forms of the same test instruments, are used.

Reference

Sparrow, S. S., Cicchetti, D. V., Saulnier, C. A., & Doll, E. A. (2016). *Vineland-3: Vineland Adaptive Behavior Scales* (3rd ed.). Psychological Corporation.

School Psychoeducational Assessment Process

The process of a school psychoeducational assessment differs from the clinical psychological or neuropsychological assessment process. The school-based process begins with educator and caregiver acknowledgement that a student is experiencing psychoeducational difficulties that persist despite mainstream teaching efforts. A Planning and Placement Team of caregivers, educators, and school-based specialists is designated and comes together to review a student's situation. As part of such a review, the Team identifies types of evaluative data that would be helpful in guiding the design of a suitable educational plan. Often, a psychoeducational assessment is included in the data requested by the Team. The formal request is made by the Team, with permission from parents or caregivers.

The school psychologist then reviews all relevant records and may elect to conduct a classroom observation in order to gain a good foundation of knowledge about the student. The student is later called out of class and asked to come to the psychologist's office for a series of test sessions. Depending on particular case needs, caregivers may also be invited to provide background information, complete behavior checklists, and respond to diagnostic interview questions. Directly with the student, the psychologist administers a relevant test battery. Since professionals in other domains are often conducting separate assessments, as requested by the Planning and Placement Team, the school psychologist's test battery tends to be more streamlined than a clinical psychological or neuropsychological test battery. Usually, the school psychoeducational test battery examines intelligence, memory, attention and concentration, developmental status, and various facets of behavioral functioning.

Once the test data are gathered and a report is written, the school psychologist consults with district colleagues and with caregivers to review the assessment findings. The Planning and Placement Team reconvenes, copies of the reports are shared, and the Team conducts a thorough discussion of all the multidisciplinary assessment findings. Based on this discussion, the Team determines the most appropriate educational approach for the designated student.

© Springer Nature Switzerland AG 2021   27
N. E. Moss, L. Moss-Racusin, *Practical Guide to Child and Adolescent Psychological Testing*, Best Practices in Child and Adolescent Behavioral Health Care, https://doi.org/10.1007/978-3-030-73515-9_5

There are several possible outcomes of Planning and Placement Team deliberations. When a student's needs are minimal, the Team may recommend continuation in a fully mainstream setting with regular education support. In some cases, a special need is recognized that can be met through relatively straightforward modifications in mainstream teaching approaches. When such modification is possible, a 504 Plan is written to authorize appropriate accommodations and take responsibility for their provision.

For some students, the evaluation findings indicate more significant needs that warrant identification as a special education student. In accord with United States federal law, the student is assigned a classification that identifies the type of special need to be addressed. The list of possible classifications is as follows: Autism, Developmental Delay, Emotional Disturbance, Hearing Impairment, Intellectual Disability, Orthopedic Impairment, Specific Learning Disabilities, Speech or Language Impairment, Traumatic Brain Injury, Visual Impairment, Other Health Impairment (Individuals with Disabilities Education Act, 2005). The Planning and Placement Team is then charged with the responsibility of writing a comprehensive, detailed Individualized Educational Plan. For students with either a 504 Plan or an Individualized Educational Plan, timely monitoring of the plan's delivery and of the student's progress is required.

Reference

Individuals with Disabilities Education Act, U.S. Department of Education § 1401-Definitions. (2005). https://uscode.house.gov/view.xhtml?path=/prelim@title20/chapter33/subchapter1&e dition=prelim

Report Interpretation

Assessment findings provide an accurate understanding of a youth and inform intervention plans. They have explanatory value that endures over many years, and they often become a benchmark against which later development is evaluated. This valuable information is summarized in the psychological assessment report. The primary goal of the test report is to convey psychological assessment findings in direct, easily accessible language that facilitates good comprehension on the part of parents and other adults charged with caring for a child or adolescent. For optimal care, it is critical that the test report become a working, much-used document, and that information contained in it be integrated into ongoing treatment plans. To be able to use psychological test results in this thorough manner, primary care providers must have a good understanding of the purpose and quality of each psychological test report section. Toward that end, each section is discussed below. The structure of psychological test reports varies somewhat across psychologists and specific types of assessments, but the components discussed below, in some form, make up the great majority of psychological test reports.

Identifying Information

This initial section of a psychological test report introduces the reader to both the youngster and to the assessment process. First, the youngster's name is provided. If a youngster does not use their given name and instead prefers a nickname or a different name altogether, it is important to refer to them throughout the report with their preferred name. However, since the report is a legal document, the youngster's legal name should be noted as such somewhere. It is most respectful to explain the appearance of a legal name ahead of time, since confusion, pain, and anger can result from being called one's non-preferred name. Sociodemographic identities

© Springer Nature Switzerland AG 2021   29
N. E. Moss, L. Moss-Racusin, *Practical Guide to Child and Adolescent
Psychological Testing*, Best Practices in Child and Adolescent Behavioral
Health Care, https://doi.org/10.1007/978-3-030-73515-9_6

may also be included in this section of the report in order to more fully understand and contextualize the youngster.

Assessment dates and the youngster's date of birth and age at the time of testing are then listed, which allows the reader to orient the assessment findings in the youngster's course of development. Additionally, calling attention to the youngster's age helps the reader begin to conceptualize appropriate expectations for someone at that specified age and developmental level. A comprehensive psychological assessment usually requires roughly 6 h of direct testing, split over a number of sessions. To maximize the validity of the test findings, lengthy intervals between the test sessions should be avoided whenever possible. Number and duration of sessions vary greatly based on a youngster's age, level of functioning, and stamina, as well as on psychologist and caregiver preferences and scheduling constraints. A few youngsters may complete their assessments in less than 6 h. Those most likely to finish quickly either feel driven to showcase their strengths by working as speedily as possible, or have very low functioning and sadly have only very modest ability or skill to demonstrate. Some youngsters, as a result of the problems that prompted their assessments, may struggle with testing and need more than the 6 h.

Grade placement is also noted, and it also helps to anchor the assessment findings in time and developmental course. In addition, the reader can see whether or not a youngster's grade placement corresponds to the normative placement for someone of their chronological age. Any lack of correspondence is clinically significant, suggesting either accelerated educational progress or academic or developmental struggles that required repetition of a grade. The school attended accompanies the grade placement information. This information is important, because it gives the reader a suggestion about the nature of the youngster's educational experience. For example, attendance at a public or private school can provide initial estimates about available special education resources (i.e., more in a public school) and class sizes (i.e., smaller in a private school). Information about school placement also indicates where to seek out educators for any necessary follow-up collaboration related to assessment findings.

Finally, psychological assessments are sometimes conducted by trainees under supervision. In such cases, the identifying information section may also include the name of the trainee's supervisor. This information is included for the sake of full transparency and also to facilitate document filing and retrieval for long after the trainee has moved on to other settings.

Background and Referral

This report section sets the foundation of the assessment. Rather than providing a global discussion of every possible aspect of the youth's history, it details the elements of the youth's development, health, professional care, and education that relate to the reason for the assessment. For example, if a high schooler is being tested to better understand poor math class performance, the background and referral section of the report should include early developmental information that speaks to fundamental capacity for academic work, as well as a description of academic skills demonstrated prior to high school. Without compromising family privacy, information is also provided about whether there is a family history that can shed light on the youth's difficulties. Also in this section, the emergence of the problems that prompted the assessment are traced, along with discussion of any earlier attempts to address the problems.

All of this documentation leads directly to the focus of the current assessment. The professional or caregiver requesting the assessment is identified, and the section then concludes with a clear statement of the specific referral questions. Thus, having reviewed this section of a good quality test report, the reader will have a succinct grasp of the origins of the problems at hand, knowledge of prior efforts to address these problems, information about the current state of the problems, and a straightforward understanding of the questions to be answered by the current assessment.

Assessment Instruments

This section lists all procedures used and formal tests administered. Test are selected based on referral questions, presenting problems, and any issues that arise during the assessment process. The function of this section is to inform the reader about the basis for the conclusions and recommendations to follow. This section should be reviewed to ensure that an adequate and relevant range of abilities, skills, behaviors, and emotions was sampled. Additionally, review of the editions used for each test is critically important. Psychological test instruments are continually revised and updated. Specifying the test edition that was used ensures that conclusions were drawn from instruments that conform to current standards for test construction and statistical rigor.

After reading the assessment instruments section of the report, the reader should have a good understanding of the justification for formulations and recommendations about the child or adolescent being assessed. The reader should also be satisfied that the utilized instruments form a relevant, acceptable basis for the conclusions drawn in the psychological assessment report.

Review of Previous Evaluations

In some cases, previous evaluation data are available. Current findings might be needed to confirm or disconfirm earlier results, resolve contradictions in prior data, track the course of a youngster's difficulties, or examine newly identified problems. Under any of these circumstances, the present data can only be interpreted accurately with the context of data obtained earlier in the youngster's development. This section provides a brief summary of each prior assessment. Such a summary should include the type of evaluation done or kind of data collected, the name of the professional who conducted the evaluation together with their credentials and any relevant institutional affiliation, the core findings, and the main recommendations. With all of this information presented in a table format, the reader of the report can efficiently acquire a great deal of critical information.

At times, caregivers or referring professionals worry that the current psychologist and assessment findings will be biased if previous evaluations are shared. With the intent of preserving objectivity, caregivers and professionals may prefer to withhold prior information until the new data are obtained. Although preservation of objectivity is an admirable goal, preventing a psychologist from reviewing past test results rarely enhances the usefulness of assessment data. Instead, requiring a psychologist to rely only on current data when prior data exist makes it impossible to do the critical work of tracing developmental patterns over the life span. In this way, fully accurate interpretation of current data is hindered. Overall, psychological testing is most useful when all available information is shared and examined.

Behavioral Observations in Assessment Setting

There are two main functions of this section of the psychological assessment report. First, the psychologist provides here a very brief description of the child or adolescent's physical appearance and mannerisms, with just enough information to allow the reader to form a mental image of the youth. Having a mental image makes the assessment data more vivid and meaningful to the reader of the report. It can also provide additional evidence for diagnostic conclusions. The description should always be written in a neutral or even complimentary tone. If the tone is critical, the reader should be concerned about broader negative bias against the youth.

Second, the psychologist describes the youngster's level of cooperation and test-taking diligence. This report section highlights any unusual features of the assessment that likely impacted the test results (e.g., unique behaviors exhibited by the youth and any particular accommodations required to facilitate their best performance). For example, a particularly frightened and angry child might climb under the assessment table and refuse to return to their chair. To accommodate them, and to avoid a power struggle and additional distress, the psychologist could choose to administer a verbal, question-and-answer test while the youngster remained under the table. Providing this information in the report informs the reader about the relative ease and comfort or lack thereof with which the youth carried out the assessment.

Based on the fulfillment of these two functions, this section concludes with guidance for the reader about how much faith to put in the findings that follow. Readers need assistance in knowing whether the reported test profile is truly representative of the youngster's current functioning or is instead an over- or underestimate of their true capacity and accomplishment.

Assessment Findings

This section is the main body of the report. Scores are reported and their meanings discussed fully. When relevant, test findings are linked to information obtained as part of the developmental history. Particular attention is paid to explaining any significant discrepancies in findings between current and previous assessments, test instruments examining similar capacities, and different areas assessed by one instrument. The youth's performance in various domains of functioning is discussed, in turn, and the relative importance of each domain in relation to the referral questions is also addressed. (Please see remaining chapters for more detailed discussion of each assessment domain.) At the conclusion of each domain discussion, the reader should look for a summary statement that offers guidance about the appropriate general conclusion to draw regarding the child or adolescent's standing in that domain. Again, language and vocabulary used should be direct and easily understood. Upon completion of reading this section of the report, the reader should have a comprehensive grasp of the youth's overall performance and a good sense of the answers to the referral questions that prompted the assessment.

Summary

In this section of the report, the most important aspects of all of the preceding sections are restated very briefly, as well as integrated. Thus, the section mentions the reasons for the assessment, the most relevant pieces of the developmental history, important features of the child or adolescent's test-taking behavior, and significant findings. This section may conclude with a precise response to the referral questions; in some reports, this task is given its own separate section.

Recommendations

Typically, the psychological assessment report concludes with a set of recommendations for how best to understand the child or adolescent and how to optimize their functioning. The recommendations flow directly from the assessment findings presented earlier in the report. To support primary care providers, parents, and caregivers in their efforts to help a child or adolescent, it is most helpful if the recommendations section begins on an encouraging note. Regardless of the level of distress about any given youth, it should always be possible to find some cause for praise related to the youth's demeanor, motivation, diligence, or capabilities. Acknowledgement of such strengths offers hope to caregivers and providers, thereby facilitating their efforts on the youngster's behalf and highlighting resiliency factors upon which they can try to build.

In regard to the recommendations, the reader should be able to identify suggestions linked to each of the problems noted in earlier report sections. Such identification is easiest for the reader if the recommendations follow the same order as the one used in the assessment instruments and assessment findings sections of the report. To illustrate, if intellectual functioning was the first domain to be reported, recommendations pertaining to intellectual functioning should come right after the encouragement discussed above.

Whenever psychological testing is carried out, the utility of reassessment should be considered. The recommendations section should end with the psychologist's best estimate of if and when reassessment would be useful. For youth receiving special education services, reassessment often adheres to timelines prescribed in educational regulations. In some cases, though, the psychologist communicates a more individualized recommendation for a particular youngster. Generally, this type of individualized recommendation is offered when monitoring of development for a specified period is required to clarify a diagnostic question, modify treatment decisions, or determine a youth's qualifications for a designated treatment or support program.

Follow-Up

In some cases, the psychological assessment findings lead very directly to further discussion with caregivers, consultation with other specialists, emergency intervention, or other case disposition. When relevant, these additional steps in caring for the youth are detailed for the reader.

Appraisal of Report Usefulness

As stressed throughout this book, primary care work in particular, as well as broader professional and personal care, can be enhanced through active application of psychological test findings. However, for anyone to be willing to take action based on psychological assessment report recommendations, they must believe that the report is valid (i.e., that the assessment was carried out in a competent manner and that the results are accurate). Certain key features are hallmarks of a valid, useful, and high quality psychological test report. They all serve an overarching purpose: to ensure that when readers finish a report, they are able to feel knowledgeable about how to help a youth, as well as empowered to do so.

First and foremost, a report should be completed in a timely manner to help ensure accuracy and utility. It should be written in clear, easily understood language; there should be an absolute minimum of technical jargon. To minimize the burden on busy readers, the report should be no longer than absolutely necessary. The assessment instruments used should be the most up-to-date editions available. They should also pertain directly to the referral questions posed. The report should be fully respectful and supportive in tone and word choice. Any unduly critical comments or negative tone should be understood as casting doubt on the validity of the report as a whole. Even if completion of the assessment proved challenging, the psychologist should be able to report the findings in an objective, instructive, and helpful manner. The report should include both the actual scores and a narrative description. Scores alone are uninterpretable for many readers; at the same time, narrative discussion without the actual scores makes it impossible to assess the accuracy of the description. Finally, there should be no mention of other youngsters. Such mention occurs occasionally when psychologists rely on a report template to maximize report-writing efficiency. Carelessness in regard to youth that are mentioned casts doubt on the trustworthiness of the data reported.

A few points related to report validity warrant particular highlighting. First, any cautionary aspects of the youngster's presentation in the testing setting should be described, and their impact on the findings should be weighed. In addition to illustrations included in the above discussion, the influence of a youngster's depression on measurement of attention and concentration, or the interference in test performance by adolescent use of non-prescription drugs, are examples of factors that could limit confidence in the testing outcomes.

Second, in reviewing the report, the reader should be able to locate responses to the specific referral questions that prompted the assessment. As stated, in some reports, these responses will be embedded in the summary discussion. In other reports, the referral questions will be explicitly repeated with accompanying responses. In either case, a good psychological test report leaves the reader clear that the original questions have been answered.

Third, it is the responsibility of the psychologist to offer relevant, helpful recommendations for a youngster, based on the assessment findings. Rather than simply repeating past or current interventions as if these were new ideas, recommendations should either offer informed support for continuation of interventions already in place or offer alternative interventions. Finally, the conclusion of a good psychological test report should give the reader guidance about how to evaluate the youngster's progress. In particular, the report should indicate if and when reassessment would be appropriate in order to gain additional, updated information.

Hopefully, the conditions outlined above are present in many psychological test reports. If a reader determines that a report falls short, though, there are two main possible steps toward obtaining much needed data. First, when possible, it is always acceptable to contact the psychologist who completed the testing for a discussion of the findings. Many times, such direct discussion can provide information that the written summary may have blurred or omitted. Second, consultation with another examiner, along with potential supplementary assessment, can often secure answers to outstanding questions about a child or adolescent.

Further Considerations

Formal Diagnosis

Although all psychological test reports discuss a range of functioning, readers will notice that reports differ in regard to provision of formal diagnosis. Some psychologists believe that psychological test data and findings are sufficient to designate specific clinical diagnoses. Other psychologists believe that without broader historical information, knowledge of family functioning, and ongoing clinical interaction, it is more justifiable to only offer comprehensive discussion of clinical functioning. Either approach can be valuable in guiding understanding and interventions.

Summary Section of Report

Before moving on to the recommendations section, many readers of psychological assessment reports choose to learn about the youngster only from the summary section. This choice is often made in the interest of efficiency and in recognition of the reader's knowledge base. While both of these considerations are legitimate, reading only the summary section of the report may leave the reader with a limited base of information. Readers who look at the full report and request any necessary clarification from the psychologist will gain the maximum benefit from psychological testing.

Commonly Encountered Scores

Results of psychological tests are expressed in the form of a variety of scores. Test authors choose among potential types of scores based on a variety of technical and statistical considerations beyond the scope of this book. To make good use of psychological test data, though, it is helpful to have a basic familiarity with the scores commonly reported in psychological test reports. The most typical scores are discussed briefly below.

Most fundamentally, the function of the test scores is to allow for comparison of the individual test-taker with a normative population of peers at the same age or grade level. Said differently, scores allow for identification of the typical range of performance on a given instrument and of when an individual test-taker places notably above or below that range. To fully grasp the normative nature of the test scores, it is critical to understand the terms mean and standard deviation. Briefly, in this context, the mean is the average score on a test; the standard deviation is the distance from the mean within which various percentages of test-takers fall.

Standard Scores

Mean = 100; standard deviation = 15. Standard scores are used most often to denote an individual's ranking in an overall population. Most Intelligence Quotient scores are reported in the form of standard scores.

Scaled Scores

Mean = 10; standard deviation = 3. Scaled scores are often used on tests of specific cognitive operations. On many psychological assessment instruments, subtest or subscale rankings are reported in the form of scaled scores, while domain-level or full-scale rankings are reported in the form of standard scores.

T-Scores

Mean = 50; standard deviation = 10. T-scores function very similarly to standard scores but with different numerical values. T-scores are used on some intelligence tests but more often on behavioral checklists and measures of developmental status.

Percentiles

Percentile scores differ from the scores discussed above in that they are not anchored around a mean score. Rather, percentile scores tell the reader the portion of the population that ranks below and above an individual test-taker on a given instrument. For example, an individual's percentile score of 89% on an intelligence test denotes that they performed better than or equal to 89% of the population. Percentile scores can be derived for a wide range of test instruments.

Age/Grade Equivalents

Age/grade equivalents identify how closely an individual test-taker's performance resembles that of a typical person of the same age or grade level. These scores are used most often on instruments that measure academic or other acquired skills. Although age/grade equivalents can be derived reliably and validly, they are often of less utility on individual psychological test reports. This reduced utility is primarily due to the enormous variation in exposure to instructive stimulation across populations.

Intelligence

Basic Definitions

Intelligence testing aims to measure innate capacity to think, reason, form judgments, make distinctions, grasp concepts, and link information in novel, original ways. Intelligence tests are typically divided into many subtests, each one measuring a specific facet of intellectual ability. The subtests are then grouped into several cognitive domains that represent broader aspects of intelligence. Finally, there is a single, summary index of the individual's overall measured intelligence.

Particular definitions of intelligence vary across measures. On some measures, intelligence is thought of as a general characteristic of an individual. This central ability is thought to determine an individual's functioning in a wide array of situations and settings. The Wechsler Scales (Wechsler, 2008, 2012, 2014) are the primary, traditional examples of tests that regard intelligence as a general, identifying factor. The series of subtests are organized into the following domains: verbal comprehension (i.e., verbal abstract reasoning, mental categorization, and the possession of factual information), perceptual organization (i.e., the ability to carry out visual-spatial analysis), fluid reasoning (i.e., flexible thinking and problem-solving), and processing speed (i.e., the efficiency with which an individual carries out cognitive tasks).

In contrast to defining intelligence as a general characteristic, intelligence may also be defined as problem-solving or mental processing ability. In other words, intelligence may consist of particular ways in which an individual manages information. This second definition of intelligence is best exemplified by the Kaufman Assessment Battery for Children (KABC-II NU; Kaufman & Kaufman, 2018). This measure examines two primary kinds of problem-solving ability, sequential and simultaneous processing. Sequential processing refers to solving problems using step-by-step, linear strategies while simultaneous processing refers to solving problems using more holistic, integrative reasoning.

© Springer Nature Switzerland AG 2021
N. E. Moss, L. Moss-Racusin, *Practical Guide to Child and Adolescent Psychological Testing*, Best Practices in Child and Adolescent Behavioral Health Care, https://doi.org/10.1007/978-3-030-73515-9_7

A short vignette provides a good illustration of these two types of basic information-processing: When asked to provide directions from their school to their home, a sequential processor responds with a series of statements such as, "Go one mile down the main road, turn right at the first traffic light, then go to the first stop sign and turn left. Go up a block and look for the house with the red door." To respond to the same request, a simultaneous processor would simply draw a map. Both ways are workable and can be successful.

The KABC-II NU (Kaufman & Kaufman, 2018) also looks at higher order mental organization and reasoning using subtests in what is termed the Planning Domain. This domain assesses the ability to manipulate information and consider anticipated developments and relationships between components and whole entities.

Taking in information is also investigated on the KABC-II NU (Kaufman & Kaufman, 2018). This investigation is carried out in the Learning and Knowledge Domains. Subtests in the Learning Domain examine immediate acquisition of novel information (i.e., how efficiently an individual can incorporate previously unknown information). Subtests in the Knowledge Domain, in contrast, measure the individual's ability to derive information from the environment over time.

Why Measure Intelligence?

Primary care providers, other professionals, parents, and caregivers are often surprised and even impatient when they learn that an intelligence test is to be part of an overall psychological test battery. Sometimes, this surprise and impatience is based on a distrust of the validity of intelligence tests, particularly in relation to members of minority groups. In fact, intelligence tests have been criticized fairly for weighting too heavily abilities, qualities, and experiences that characterize the dominant cultural group or race while failing to assess equally important characteristics and attributes more characteristic of minority groups (Suzuki et al., 2001). While such criticism has merit, contemporary editions of intelligence tests have reduced these contaminants and biases. Furthermore, with proper interpretation of intelligence test findings (e.g., careful integration of them with history, observations, and results on other test instruments), critical information about an individual can be obtained.

In other cases, question about the need for an intelligence measure is based on the assumption that an individual's difficulties can be fully understood by focusing solely on observable behaviors, specific acquired skills (i.e., not innate ability), and emotions, without attention to their intellectual capacity. However, to be interpreted accurately, an individual's behaviors, performance on tests of skills, and emotions must be understood in the context of intellectual endowment. Intelligence test results allow examiners and all those involved with a youngster to understand what is fair to expect of them.

Identical observations of a youngster should be interpreted differently depending on intelligence level. For example, a boy hospitalized in a psychiatric unit may be noted to be repeating "Why?" as he goes through his day. This behavior is first interpreted by the staff as an emotional expression of confusion and despair. Intelligence testing then reveals that the youngster has a severe Intellectual Disability. Additional consultation with his previous special educators indicates that he had been taught a simple sorting task (i.e., separating into piles the cardboard cutouts of letters in his name). His name ended in "Y." What had been interpreted as a social-emotional plea was actually a fixation on a very concrete bit of experience. He was not saying "Why?" He was, instead, repeating "Y." Without the intelligence test findings, the staff would have focused their efforts at a level way beyond this youngster's developmental capacity, thereby leaving his needs unmet. With the intelligence test findings, the staff can provide appropriate redirection and new instruction. While this case represents a very extreme discrepancy between conclusions based on clinical observation versus assessment findings, many less extreme cases reflect equally impactful contrasts.

Overall, intelligence measures anchor interpretation of an entire test battery. The information yielded by intelligence testing about a youngster's intellectual capacity helps to promote an accurate understanding of the youngster and to guide a variety of interventions on their behalf. For example, intelligence data support diagnostic precision and eligibility for program participation. More deeply, intelligence test results help to characterize the fundamental nature of an individual's way of thinking. The nature of an individual's thought varies according to innate capacities for grasping abstract, comprehensive concepts versus needing concrete, specific facts; for managing complexity versus needing simplicity; and for displaying flexibility versus needing rigid rules. These characteristic capacities help to determine what seems important or even interesting to an individual, what they can accept as evidence for a point of view, how they can formulate plans, and the extent to which they can sustain efforts aimed at implementation of those plans.

Furthermore, given the nature of their variability, these capacities dictate which approaches to an individual are likely to be understood and accepted most easily. For successful, cooperative action, information should be communicated in a style that is congruent with the individual's level of intelligence. Likewise, an individual's responses can be interpreted most accurately if understood in the correct intellectual context. Communication in ways that are inconsistent with an individual's intellectual level result only in frustration, irritation, a sense of being misunderstood, and an unwillingness to cooperate.

Attunement to intellectual level is most acutely necessary when caring for individuals with limited intellectual ability. Among compassionate, dedicated caregivers and providers, there is often a well-intentioned but misguided reluctance to acknowledge a youth's cognitive limitations. This reluctance is rooted in a wish to avoid behaving in ways that could be labeled as rude, insulting, and minimizing or even limiting of the youth's abilities. As a result, caregivers and providers may speak and relate at a level way beyond the youngster's capacity. While some youth will make their confusion clear (e.g., by acting out in the form of oppositional or disruptive behavior), many more will outwardly appear to be in quiet agreement with the communication. However, their internal confusion will prevent appropriate follow-up cooperation. The kindest approach to individuals is to respect both their inborn strengths and limitations so that much needed care can be provided precisely, appropriately, and helpfully, and without undue pressure that can painfully assault their self-esteem.

The importance of adjusting to an individual's level of intelligence has particular relevance for primary care providers. Primary care providers often have to synthesize a great deal of data, conceptualize a treatment plan, and then convey that plan to a patient and their caregivers. The plan's utility and the likelihood of it being pursued depend greatly on how well patients can understand the material presented to them and enact what is being asked of them. Their understanding and follow through, in turn, depend to a great extent on the goodness-of-fit between the plan, how it is presented, and their own intellectual capacity to grasp information.

Primary care providers can serve their patients well and minimize their own frustration by mastering the information offered below about how thought differs and about which approaches have the most potential for success at various intelligence levels. Although children and adolescents rarely have full responsibility for interacting with medical professionals – parents and caregivers typically mediating that interaction – young patients still deserve to understand their situations and proposed treatments. Furthermore, youngsters' cooperation is crucial for successful implementation of adults' plans. Thus, grasping the way a young patient thinks, and relating to them appropriately, can make a critical difference in quality of care. Additionally, while data about caregivers' intelligence levels are usually unavailable and beyond the scope of pediatric primary care, the recommendations presented below may also facilitate successful communication with caregivers of young patients.

Common Patterns of Difficulty

Intelligence Quotient = 140+, Very Superior

Nature of Thought Individuals at this highest level of intelligence truly think and understand the world in ways that are beyond most everyone at lower intelligence levels. They grasp intricacies and abstractions that most people cannot comprehend. Connections between ideas, processes, and objects are clear to them while outside others' awareness. Importantly, individuals at this highest level of intelligence are significantly better than individuals at lower intelligence levels at noting the implications of events and concepts and then formulating appropriate, relevant expectations and plans. With appropriate support and understanding, development of intellectual abilities at this level can be absolutely exhilarating.

A potential difficulty for these highly intelligent individuals is that they sometimes struggle with the fact that other people really cannot match their intellectual capacity. At times, when they underestimate the difference between their intellectual acumen and that of others, these highly intelligent individuals can become severely frustrated. When the gulf between their intelligence and that of others is more accurately perceived but not bridged, individuals with very superior intelligence can become lonely and isolated. Another potential difficulty for children and adolescents with very superior intelligence is that their high level thought may confuse their peers and threaten their teachers, parents, and caregivers. At times, their comments and behavior can be misinterpreted as challenging or oppositional when, in actuality, they are merely operating at a higher than expected intellectual level. Additionally, insufficiently challenging educational experiences can bore and frustrate these youngsters. Their interests may also be out of sync with those of their agemates.

Despite the challenges, very superior intellectual endowment opens up a rich, stimulating world of knowledge and ideas. In addition, it is often the case that when youngsters in this intelligence range are diagnosed with coexisting mental disorders, their impressive intelligence can be a very helpful resource in coping. For example, an extremely bright youngster on the Autism Spectrum can likely understand that they have a lifelong disorder impacting their social functioning. They can likely also further understand that conflict with others often relates to their fundamental social impairment, and that learning specific social skills will lessen their discomfort and promote their acceptance by others.

How Do We Help? When interacting with youths at the very superior level of intelligence, adults should be prepared to listen a great deal. By following as closely as possible the youth's statements and by attending to their nonverbal communication (i.e., facial expressions, tone of voice, posture, body movements, etc.), the adult can identify points at which to intervene with support. Supportive intervention can take the form of encouragement and validation. For the best results, it is helpful to communicate using an appropriately sophisticated vocabulary.

In situations relevant to the practice of primary care, intervention may need to include acceptance and exploration of the patient's intellectual or philosophical analysis of relevant medical issues and treatment-planning. The intervention may then need to take the form of redirecting the youngster's attention to specific problems or issues that require particular action. Generally, adult interaction with youngsters at the very superior intelligence level will be the most useful if the adult seeks to make clear the ways in which other people may not understand the youngster or see situations with the same clarity that is apparent to the youngster. The adult can then suggest behaviors that will facilitate better understanding from others and, specifically within the practice of primary care, promote a better medical outcome for the youngster.

Intelligence Quotient = 130–139, Very Superior

Nature of Thought Much of the above discussion about the nature of thought in individuals with intelligence scores of 140 and above applies to individuals with scores in the 130's, as well. Individuals in this range of intelligence display easy mastery of abstractions and higher order concepts. Their reasoning abilities are extremely impressive. They are interested in philosophical and intellectual questions that arise from day-to-day interactions and communication of information. The primary difference between individuals at this level and those at the intellectual level above them is that, while they are very bright, they tend to think in ways that are more familiar to the broader population. Their intellectual outlook is not as fundamentally different from the mainstream as that of the individuals with intelligence scores of 140 and above.

How Do We Help? Again, much of what is helpful with the individuals in the highest intelligence range is also helpful with individuals in this range. Discussion of the subtle nuances of situations and of the complexities of subjects is satisfying and reassuring to individuals at this high level of intellectual ability.

For primary care providers treating children and adolescents in this range of intelligence, it is important to be prepared to discuss a patient's medical status as fully as they request. Providers should acknowledge the patient's capacity to grasp complex medical information and to comprehend even complicated medical treatment-planning. Thoughtful, high level discussion paired with sensitive attention to a youngster's emotional reactions offers the best chance for good patient cooperation and successful treatment outcomes.

Intelligence Quotient = 120–129, Superior

Nature of Thought Individuals in the superior range of intelligence are quite bright. They can master abstractions and generalizations. They display good reasoning ability and can follow intricate lines of thought. Given a specific piece of information, they can think comfortably about its implications and consequences. They can design plans of action that derive appropriately from specific information. However, unlike individuals at even higher intelligence levels, they may reach the limits of their understanding a bit sooner.

How Do We Help? For individuals with intelligence scores in the 120's, it is best to recognize their strong intellectual ability. Discussion of nuances and complexity is useful and can be carried out with a reasonably sophisticated vocabulary. In mild contrast to their higher level peers, though, they often need slightly more intellectual support to identify connections among ideas. They benefit more often from clarification of ideas and from guidance in designing plans of action.

Within the context of primary care, barring other psychological or emotional limitations, patients at this intelligence level have little trouble grasping medical information and cooperating with their care. Diagnostic information can be conveyed fully, just as treatment plans can be laid out with well-founded hope that they will be accepted and implemented. However, primary care providers should still be alert to these patients' possible unique misunderstandings or lapses in comprehension (e.g., simple confusion of vocabulary terms, more concern than necessary in response to medical information), providing explanation and reorientation as necessary.

It is important to note here that individuals with superior and very superior intellect are rare in the overall population. Even skilled medical professionals may not have such unusual intelligence levels. Still, when children and adolescents with these outstanding intellects present for primary care, it remains critically important to align treatment interventions with their high intellectual level. This sort of alignment can be challenging for providers, particularly in those instances when a young patient's intelligence may be higher than theirs. Young patients may seem intentionally intimidating or insulting to providers. In such difficult moments, it is useful to maintain the perspective that these patients are still children or adolescents. No matter how bright they are, they cannot possibly yet have the experience, wisdom, and judgment possessed by their elders. With this perspective, it becomes more possible to provide the information and reassurance that young patients need badly in order to be able to benefit most from medical care.

Intelligence Quotient = 110–119, High Average

Nature of Thought In the high average range of intelligence, individuals display an easy understanding of factual knowledge. They can categorize and retain information. They can comprehend, process, and respond to thoughtfully presented information, bringing their own prior experience to bear. They are comfortable following clear directions. Abstractions and generalizations are meaningful to individuals at this level of intelligence, especially when explained thoroughly. Given these abilities, interactions with individuals at this level of intelligence may suggest that they can function at an even higher level. Believing that they possess greater capacity than they actually have, others may expect these individuals to be able to engage in highly creative, original thought, linking novel information with sophisticated conceptualizations. Unfortunately, such expectations are frequently unmet, not due to any wish to frustrate other people, but rather to the basic nature of this level of intellectual ability.

How Do We Help? For individuals with intelligence scores between 110 and 119, it is most productive to engage in clear, informative conversation. Facts should be stated in a straightforward manner, and examples should be offered to support the information conveyed. A variety of consequences and implications deriving from the presented facts should be set forth and discussed. Possible directions for further thought or action should be suggested. Individuals at this intelligence level will likely need some repetition and clarification in order to fully consolidate the information that is conveyed to them. Guidance may also be helpful to enhance their own expression of their knowledge.

In line with this framework about how to relate to individuals with high average intelligence, primary care providers working with them should lay out medical data in a clear, well-organized manner. Patients should be walked through information so that they do not have to rely solely on their own abilities to process the information. Treatment plans should be spelled out in vocabulary that is readily understandable. When clearly invited to, patients at this level of intellectual ability can be expected to be able to raise necessary questions and concerns.

Intelligence Quotient = 100–109, Average

Nature of Thought People with this average level of intelligence have a solid understanding of concrete, factual information. Categories of knowledge are meaningful to them, although manipulating and linking these categories is often quite challenging. High level abstractions and generalizations are of little interest to most people at this intelligence level. They tend to think in fairly uncomplicated, straightforward ways. Often, they need to review information to feel a sufficient sense of mastery and comfort. Even more often, they need others to explicitly identify the implications of information being discussed. Without such explicit guidance, individuals at this level of intelligence often become frustrated. For them, communication of higher level ideas without translation into concrete action steps is interpreted as incomplete assistance, at best, and as an intentional effort to withhold essential help, at worst.

How Do We Help? To relate well to individuals with intelligence scores between 100 and 109, it is best to engage in down to earth, uncomplicated discussion. The focus should be on specific, concrete problems and how to solve them. With guidance and reassurance, it is reasonable to expect that individuals at this level will respond well to requests for measured cognitive flexibility. However, significant originality in their thought should not be expected.

For primary care providers, two aspects of treatment are most important with patients at this level of intelligence. First, to maximize patient comfort and treatment compliance, it is necessary to provide a full discussion of all relevant facts. This discussion should move at a methodical pace and provide ample opportunity for questions. Second, in regard to treatment compliance specifically, substantial prediction and guidance should be provided regarding any expected choice points or steps at which the patient might have to evaluate their condition and make a decision about how to proceed. Individuals at this level of intellectual capacity can follow this type of guidance but tend to have trouble generating their own ideas about an appropriate plan of action.

Intelligence Quotient = 90–99, Average

Nature of Thought Individuals with intelligence scores in the 90's are capable of learning much of a typical academic curriculum and can master a wide range of skills needed for vocational success. At the same time, their intellectual capacity dictates that they think in very concrete terms. Repetitive procedures, highly specific illustrations of relevant issues, and clear instructions are much more meaningful and convincing for them than abstractions or broad rationales. Furthermore, once rules and schedules are learned, it is very difficult for an individual with intelligence in the 90–99 range to feel comfortable with any deviation, no matter how reasonable such a deviation might seem to others.

How Do We Help? Interactions with individuals in this intelligence range can go smoothly as long as the individuals' needs for predictability, concrete explanations, and clear expectations are accommodated. The individual's comfort with readily understood material should be respected; ideas and issues should be discussed in concrete terms. Communication should be direct and limited to the most important topics to be managed. Repetition is helpful. Requests for cognitive and behavioral flexibility should be kept to a minimum. If change in a plan or routine becomes essential, guidance should be offered in the form of teaching a new concrete set of rules to replace the previously acquired set.

In the primary care setting, it is most important to accommodate to a person's average intellectual level when conveying diagnostic information and when outlining a treatment plan. To be best understood by an individual with an intelligence score in the 90's, diagnostic information should be discussed in brief, straightforward, declarative sentences. Diagnoses should be linked directly to observable symptoms. Similarly, in presenting a treatment plan, the emphasis should be on clear, concrete instructions regarding procedures and medication compliance, if relevant. Intervention strategies should also be linked directly to observable symptoms. Step-by-step directions should be offered about desirable actions in the event of a treatment plan disruption. Additionally, for productive provider-patient relationships, it is critical that the provider interpret a patient's struggles with flexibility as, at least in part, a reflection of intellectual constraints rather than as oppositionality or resistance.

Intelligence Quotient = 80–89, Low Average

Nature of Difficulty Individuals in this intelligence range have more limited intelligence. While they also can learn academically and gain marketable skills, they operate on a simpler level and generally at a slower pace than individuals at higher intelligence levels. For people with intelligence scores in the 80's, much of their intellectual activity involves exerting effort to grasp simple, basic ideas. Often, they must check and re-check to be sure that their understanding is correct. They also devote a great deal of thought to how to obtain desired objects and situational outcomes. Individuals with low average intelligence are easily confused by too much detail and extraneous information. In many instances, an individual in this intelligence range may correctly latch onto one detail but misinterpret its relevance and implications; such misunderstandings can lead to uncomfortable disagreements.

How Do We Help? When interacting with individuals in the 80–89 intelligence range, it is best to be very clear and soothing. Ample explanations should be offered for any necessary action. It is essential, though, that these explanations be delivered using extremely simple vocabulary. Communication should proceed slowly and with many opportunities for illustration and explicit guidance. Very concrete problem-solving strategies should be taught. Moreover, continuing guidance is essential for optimal performance.

The self-reports of young patients in the low average intelligence range can, for the most part, be considered generally accurate. However, patient capacity to ask relevant questions and to accurately process the answers to those questions constitutes a key issue for primary care providers working with youngsters with low average intellect. While it is generally considered best to give patients the chance to raise questions about their treatment and to receive informative answers, individuals with intelligence scores in the 80's tend to have a hard time formulating appropriate questions and to misunderstand central aspects of their illness and care. Providers themselves should ask sufficient questions to accurately gauge their patient's grasp of relevant information.

Patients at this intelligence level could easily feel more panic and apprehension about medical treatment procedures than would be experienced by their more intelligent peers. Within the domain of primary care, it is very important to recognize and work to reduce this discomfort. At the same time, individuals at this intelligence level might fail to appreciate the larger implications of their medical issues. In such cases, the patients might actually experience less than reasonable distress in the face of serious diagnoses and medical treatment regimens that require careful, timed precision. In these cases, primary care providers should carefully weigh the individual risks and benefits involved in the patient more fully grasping the seriousness of their situation.

Intelligence Quotient = 70–79, Borderline

Nature of Difficulty Engaging in cognitive activity is very difficult for people with intelligence scores in the 70's. Individuals at this level have limited cognitive ability. They grasp very simple ideas and behavioral sequences. When interpersonally comfortable, they may focus on particular pieces of information and mimic the actions of individuals around them. Also in comfortable situations, they may display enjoyment and some appreciation for humor, which can give the impression that they have greater intellectual ability than they actually possess. In fact, thought is extremely concrete and simplistic for individuals in the borderline range of intelligence.

How Do We Help? For optimal interactions with individuals in this intelligence range, care providers should keep all transactions at a markedly slow pace. Using a basic vocabulary, communication should be very simple. Explanations and instructions should be brief. Every effort should be made to make directions extremely easy to understand. Multi-step instructions should be avoided in favor of clear, concrete, single-step instructions. Easy-to-master routines should be suggested and modeled. Multiple repetitions of important information should be provided.

For primary care providers working with youngsters at this level of intelligence, it is possible to rely on patient self-report as an accurate symptom index. However, verification from parents or caregivers would be appropriate. Additionally, it is important to be vigilant to youngsters in this intelligence range potentially misunderstanding key information, fixating on specific aspects of their illness or treatment, and suffering unwarranted distress. With attentiveness and quick intervention, such misunderstanding can be prevented or at least minimized, allowing for more optimal participation in medical care.

Intelligence Quotient = 60–69, Mild Intellectual Disability

Nature of Difficulty Provided they have impaired adaptive functioning, individuals in this intelligence range are considered intellectually disabled. Their thinking is extremely simple and concrete. They can acquire specific cognitive and behavioral associations. However, even when seemingly reasonable and easily managed, requests for flexibility or modifications in these associations are extremely confusing and distressing. Individuals with mild Intellectual Disability may identify goals or wishes, and they may also insist on fulfillment of these desires. However, they often have no understanding of the necessary steps to meet their goals. Many times, since they typically cannot grasp the nature of their limitations, they see other people as obstacles to their satisfaction. This misunderstanding of others' behavior can lead to anger and discord.

How Do We Help? The techniques described above for relating to individuals in the borderline intellectual range are all applicable to individuals with mild Intellectual Disability, as well. In light of the latter's greater impairment, though, the techniques should be extended and intensified for them. All communication and instruction should be simplified greatly. A very slow pace is essential for understanding. Efforts should focus on teaching basic skills that facilitate everyday life.

In primary care practice, providers are likely to be most successful if they relate in a warm, friendly, and supportive manner; focus on reassuring the patient about their safety and wellbeing; and frame medical information in the most elementary of terms. Although patients in this intelligence range can directly manifest their emotional state and level of physical discomfort, the provider should rely on parents and caregivers to convey, receive, and manage critical information about symptomatology and treatment-planning.

Intelligence Quotient = Below 60, Mild/Moderate/Severe/
Profound Intellectual Disability (Committee to Evaluate
the Supplemental Security Income Disability Program
for Children with Mental Disorders et al., 2015)

Nature of Difficulty Thinking becomes increasingly difficult with each more significant level of cognitive impairment. Individuals in this intelligence range have a profound focus on the present moment, without ability to consider impacts and consequences. Actions are taken without thought and reflection. Behavioral routines, with the guidance of more capable individuals, are most important. In many cases, individuals with these more impactful intellectual disabilities also struggle with multiple physical ailments and unusual anatomical features; the fundamental sources of impairment often do not only impact intellectual functioning but physical functioning and medical status, as well. Comorbid conditions and cognitive impairments can then each intensify the impact of the other.

How Do We Help? Individuals with intelligence scores below 60 require considerable and often massive assistance and care. Primary care providers, along with all others interacting with these individuals, should share critical information with parents and caregivers. Intervention efforts, when possible, should emphasize instruction in life skills and adaptive behavior. Along with basic medical data, a patient's nonverbal behavior (i.e., facial expressions, vocalizations, body posturing, etc.), should be monitored as an index of patient comfort and intervention success.

Prominent Instruments

The Woodcock-Johnson Tests of Cognitive Abilities (WJ IV COG; Schrank et al., 2014) are an alternative to both the Wechsler Scales (Wechsler, 2008, 2012, 2014) and the KABC-II NU (Kaufman & Kaufman, 2018), both described above. This test is quite comprehensive, as it includes measures of both fundamental intelligence, defined as a multi-faceted, underlying attribute of an individual, as well as scholastic accomplishments. Similar in structure to other intelligence measures, the test battery is composed of numerous subtests grouped into relevant cognitive domains.

Many school districts rely heavily on the WJ IV COG (Schrank et al., 2014) for school-based assessments. The subtests' focus and the instrument's breadth appear to facilitate incorporation of the test data into academic program-planning. In more clinical settings, psychologists working with children and adolescents often use specific subtests, as opposed to the entire battery, to probe more deeply into particular areas of functioning. Information obtained in this way helps to confirm or disconfirm interpretive hypotheses raised by findings on different instruments (Table 1).

Table 1 Prominent instruments for assessing intelligence

Test name and publication date	Age range	Information provided by test
Wechsler Preschool and Primary Scale of Intelligence – Fourth Edition (WPPSI-IV) 2012	2 years, 6 months – 7 years, 7 months	2 years, 6 months – 3 years, 11 months: Verbal comprehension Visual spatial Working memory Vocabulary acquisition Nonverbal General ability
		4 years, 0 months – 7 years, 7 months: Verbal comprehension Visual spatial Fluid reasoning Working memory Processing speed Vocabulary acquisition Nonverbal General ability Cognitive proficiency
Wechsler Intelligence Scale for Children – Fifth Edition (WISC-V) 2014	6 years, 0 months – 16 years, 11 months	Verbal comprehension Visual spatial Fluid reasoning Working memory Processing speed Quantitative reasoning Auditory working memory Nonverbal General ability Cognitive proficiency Expanded (verbal expanded crystallized, expanded fluid) Naming speed Symbol translation Storage and retrieval
Wechsler Adult Intelligence Scale – Fourth Edition (WAIS-IV) 2008	16 years, 0 months – 90 years, 11 months	Verbal comprehension Perceptual reasoning Working memory Processing speed
Kaufman Assessment Battery for Children – Second Editions Normative Update (KABC-II NU) 2018	3 years – 18 years	Simultaneous Sequential Planning Learning Knowledge

(continued)

Table 1 (continued)

Test name and publication date	Age range	Information provided by test
Woodcock-Johnson IV Tests of Cognitive Abilities (WJ IV COG) 2014	2 years – 90+ years	General intellectual ability Brief intellectual ability Fluid reasoning and comprehension-knowledge composite Comprehension-knowledge Fluid reasoning Short-term working memory Cognitive processing speed Auditory processing Long-term retrieval Visual processing Quantitative reasoning Auditory memory span Number facility Perceptual speed Vocabulary Cognitive efficiency

References

Committee to Evaluate the Supplemental Security Income Disability Program for Children with Mental Disorders, Board on the Health of Select Populations, Board on Children, Youth, and Families, Institute of Medicine, Division of Behavioral and Social Sciences and Education, & The National Academics of Sciences, Engineering, and Medicine. (2015). *Mental disorders and disabilities among low-income children* (T. F. Boat & J. T. Wu, Eds.). National Academies Press.

Kaufman, A. S., & Kaufman, N. L. (2018). *KABC-II NU: Kaufman Assessment Battery for Children* (2nd ed., Normative Update). Pearson, Psychological Corporation.

Schrank, F. A., McGrew, K. S., & Mather, N. (2014). *Woodcock-Johnson IV Tests of Cognitive Abilities* (4th ed.). Riverside.

Suzuki, L. A., Ponterotto, J. G., & Meller, P. J. (2001). *Handbook of multicultural assessment: Clinical, psychological, and educational applications* (L. A. Suzuki, J. G. Ponterotto, & P. J. Meller, Eds., 2nd ed.). Jossey-Bass.

Wechsler, D. (2008). *WAIS-IV: Wechsler Adult Intelligence Scale* (4th ed.). Psychological Corporation.

Wechsler, D. (2012). *WPPSI-IV: Wechsler Preschool and Primary Scale of Intelligence* (4th ed.). Pearson, Psychological Corporation.

Wechsler, D. (2014). *WISC-V: Wechsler Intelligence Scale for Children* (5th ed.). NCS Pearson, Inc.

Speech and Language

Basic Definitions

Assessment in this domain examines an individual's skill with oral and written language. In regard to oral communication, testing focuses on the mechanics of speech, as well as the understanding and instrumental use of language (receptive and expressive language, respectively). In regard to written communication, test instruments examine recognition and usage of spelling, grammar and punctuation, and meaningful self-expression. In addition, speech-language assessment focuses on pragmatic language (i.e., the more concrete, practical language skills necessary to engage successfully in daily interactions). Making requests, responding to questions, or taking turns in a conversation are important examples of pragmatic language.

Why Measure Speech and Language?

Examining speech-language skills from a psychological perspective allows for confirmation or disconfirmation of communication skills as the source of the difficulties that prompt an assessment. It is important to know whether concerns about a youngster reflect underlying deficits across domains or a primary difficulty with communicating needs, wants, strengths, and weaknesses. When scores on speech-language instruments are equivalent to most other cognitive test scores, a speech-language disorder is unlikely to be a core element in a youngster's difficulty. In contrast, when speech-language test scores are quite low and/or different from associated scores, concern is justified about a significant communication disorder. For those cases in which speech-language functioning is less central, the psychological test report should direct the reader to the appropriate source of

© Springer Nature Switzerland AG 2021   53
N. E. Moss, L. Moss-Racusin, *Practical Guide to Child and Adolescent Psychological Testing*, Best Practices in Child and Adolescent Behavioral Health Care, https://doi.org/10.1007/978-3-030-73515-9_8

difficulties and any necessary interventions. In cases in which speech-language functioning appears to play a pivotal role, it is best to refer the youth for more in-depth testing by a speech-language specialist.

In regard to the speech and language domain, psychological assessment findings should be conceptualized as serving a screening function. Clinical psychologists are well-trained to administer measures that provide basic data related to communication conditions. However, more precise diagnosis of, and treatment-planning for, a speech-language disorder is beyond psychologists' expertise. Again, when psychological test data identify a marked difficulty with speech-language functioning, it is most appropriate to refer a youngster for more comprehensive evaluation by a speech-language specialist. For many youngsters, particularly very young children, formal speech-language therapy will then be indicated. When provided by skilled professionals, such therapy is extremely beneficial.

While further evaluation and specialized treatment are often required, there are also helpful steps that can be taken based solely on psychological test findings. For example, it is important that primary care providers, parents, caregivers, and teachers be informed of a youngster's speech-language condition. When well informed, adults can be most appropriate both in their interpretation of a youngster's communication style, and also in their communication approach to a given youngster. Most critically, adults need to refrain from interpreting a youngster's behavior as willfully difficult when it may simply be a manifestation of a communication problem.

Common Patterns of Difficulty

Receptive Language Better Than Expressive Language

Nature of Difficulty For some individuals, their understanding of communication from others surpasses their facility with expressing themselves. Poor self-expression can manifest as having marked difficulty with answering questions, conveying needs, or explaining oneself to others.

Such a profile can signify a variety of underlying conditions. Most optimistically, this skill pattern is often seen in young children who are beginning to communicate verbally. It is not atypical for youngsters to comprehend speech before they can produce it themselves (Grimm et al., 2011). Thus, in young children, better receptive than expressive language may simply be an index of unfolding development. In older children and adolescents, comparatively weaker expressive language skills are more often manifestations of some level of disorder. In some cases, this disorder is an impairment in language development. In other cases, the poorer expressive skills are an aspect of a broader developmental disorder (e.g., Intellectual Disability or Autism Spectrum Disorder).

How Do We Help? For youngsters whose receptive language is better than their expressive language, adults should use every naturally occurring opportunity to introduce and explain new vocabulary words. Adults should also use the same sort of opportunities to demonstrate and elucidate verbal exchanges. Daily interaction provides many chances to practice supported oral self-expression.

Expressive Language Better Than Receptive Language

Nature of Difficulty In contrast to the pattern described above, assessment data sometimes indicate that an individual's self-expression ranks at a higher level than their actual understanding of verbal communication. For such an individual, expressive facility tends to be superficial, even when manifested in ample verbal output and a large vocabulary. This superficial verbal fluency masks the underlying impaired understanding. Individuals with this score profile seem to know more than they actually do grasp. Inappropriate behavior and confusing and/or aggravating responses are often signs of underlying problems with receptive language.

How Do We Help? In relation to youngsters whose expressive language is better than their receptive language, primary care providers, parents, caregivers, and teachers should always check to ensure that the youngsters actually understand what is conveyed to them. This is particularly important if a youngster's behavior seems out of line with what has been said to them. Again, for these youngsters, verbal facility cannot be reliably trusted as an accurate gauge for basic comprehension.

Generalized Communication Problem

Nature of Difficulty Some youngsters score poorly on tests of cognitive ability despite giving the informal impression of possessing better intelligence. At times, these youngsters are performing poorly, because impaired general management of language prevents them from displaying their full abilities. Trouble finding just the right word to use; speaking in roundabout, circumstantial patterns; or fundamentally not knowing how to put thoughts into words are all possible signals of a more comprehensive communication disorder.

How Do We Help? To arrive at an accurate diagnostic understanding and then to make a useful treatment plan, it is essential to distinguish accurately between communication difficulties and compromised intellectual ability. As is written above, children and adolescents displaying broad communication problems should be referred for specialized speech-language evaluations.

Impaired Pragmatic Language and Unusual Prosody

Nature of Difficulty As a reminder, pragmatic language refers to all of the practical communication skills necessary to negotiate smooth social interactions. Some of these skills are verbal (e.g., making requests, offering explanations, and conversational turn-taking), while others are nonverbal (e.g., facial expressions, tone of voice, and use of gestures). Individuals with problematic pragmatic language have significant struggles with interpersonal interaction, often resulting in disrupted social transactions. For example, an adolescent with impaired pragmatic language skills might blow up at a store cashier because of difficulty negotiating a plan to deal with the lack of availability of a desired item.

Prosody, a distinct but related construct to pragmatic language, refers to the sound patterns involved in speech (i.e., rhythm, intonations, volume, and rate). While difficulties with prosody can be measured formally, they are also readily apparent in even informal interactions. Problems with prosody are often quite striking. Listeners are often uncomfortable with an affected individual's communication and may have to strain to understand that individual. Most often, problems with pragmatic language and poor prosody are associated with major developmental difficulties, particularly Autism Spectrum Disorder.

How Do We Help? To be effective, assistance with pragmatic language and unusual prosody typically must be delivered by professionals with highly specialized training. This assistance should be conceptualized as part of speech-language therapy and social skills instruction.

Single Word Vocabulary Better Than Fuller Language Usage

Nature of Difficulty In some youngsters, there is a marked contrast between robust knowledge of single words and capacity to use that vocabulary in meaningful verbal communication. Furthermore, these youngsters may have difficulty linking (albeit impressive) isolated words into more complex communication.

How Do We Help? For these youngsters, it is important to resist being misled by the relatively better scores on tests that measure only vocabulary size. Additionally, as with individuals experiencing pragmatic language and prosody problems, speech-language specialists are often the best equipped to help these youngsters transform their single word vocabulary into broader communication skills. It is also true that language-rich environments can be very useful in promoting communication development. Primary care providers can help their patients by encouraging the adults in their patients' lives to model verbal exchange and to engage children and adolescents in ample conversation.

Speech Production

Nature of Difficulty At times, both assessment findings and behavioral observations during testing highlight specific difficulties with aspects of producing speech. These difficulties include disfluency (i.e., trouble getting words out smoothly or disruptions in speaking), misarticulation (i.e., problems with proper use of the bodily organs involved in the production of speech), and incorrect pronunciation of words (i.e., errors in vocalizing the sounds associated with particular letters or in appropriately emphasizing certain syllables). All of these speech production difficulties can interfere with interpersonal communication and may eventually lead to impaired self-esteem.

How Do We Help? For youngsters who experience severe trouble with speech production, therapy with a speech-language pathologist is most often essential. In addition, a referral for an assistive technology evaluation can be very useful. (See Visual-Motor Coordination chapter for further information about such an evaluation.) Assistive technology often includes devices to augment or replace an individual's own production of the spoken word.

Prominent Instruments

It is important to distinguish between a full speech-language assessment and examination of speech-language functioning as part of a psychological test battery. Speech pathologists have a wealth of well-standardized instruments on which to draw in pursuing an in-depth, detailed understanding of a youth's communication capacities and skills. Using these instruments, communication experts are able to provide specialized guidance regarding appropriate interventions related to speech-language functioning. In contrast, psychologists seek to determine how speech-language functioning compares to a youth's functioning in other developmental domains. To this end, psychologists tend to utilize a few primary instruments to sample speech-language capacities and skills. These instruments typically use pictorial and written prompts, a fill-in-the blank format, and vocabulary lists.

The Peabody Picture Vocabulary Test (PPVT-5; Dunn, 2018) is a common instrument used in psychological test batteries. The test measures a youth's understanding of spoken words at the single word level. Well-standardized, long-used, and widely accepted for use with children and adolescents, the test indicates the level of a youth's most basic receptive vocabulary.

Often administered in tandem with the PPVT-5 (Dunn, 2018), the Expressive Vocabulary Test (EVT-3; Williams, 2018) is a widely used measure of a child or adolescent's skill at calling up correct words to label objects in the environment and make themselves understood by others. Findings on the EVT-3 (Williams, 2018) relate primarily to simple use of language (i.e., expressive vocabulary).

Table 1 Prominent instruments for assessing speech and language

Test name and publication date	Age range	Information provided by test
Peabody Picture Vocabulary Test – Fifth Edition (PPVT-5) 2018	2 years, 6 months – 90+ years	Receptive vocabulary
Expressive Vocabulary Test – Third Edition (EVT-3) 2018	2 years, 6 months – 90+ years	Expressive vocabulary
Oral and Written Language Scales, Second Edition (OWLS-II) 2011	3 years, 0 months – 21 years, 11 months for listening comprehension and oral expression	Scales: Listening comprehension Oral expression Reading comprehension Written expression
	5 years, 0 months – 21 years, 11 months for reading comprehension and written expression	Each scale assesses linguistic structures: Lexical/semantic Syntactic Pragmatic Supralinguistic

While the PPVT-5 (Dunn, 2018) and the EVT-3 (Williams, 2018) focus mainly on basic vocabulary, the Oral and Written Language Scales (OWLS-II; Carrow-Woolfolk, 2011) examine broader speech-language functioning. They address oral language in relation to both receptive (i.e., Listening Comprehension Scale) and expressive (i.e., Oral Expression Scale) communication, along with both the comprehension of written language (i.e., Reading Comprehension Scale) and the actual use of written language (i.e., Written Expression Scale). Data generated from the OWLS-II (Carrow-Woolfolk, 2011) allow the psychologist to go beyond examination of basic vocabulary to examination of the youth's facility with more complex communication (Table 1).

References

Carrow-Woolfolk, E. (2011). *OWLS-II: Oral and Written Language Scales* (2nd ed.). Western Psychological Services.
Dunn, D. M. (2018). *Peabody Picture Vocabulary Test* (5th ed.). NCS Pearson.
Grimm, A., Müller, A., Hamann, C., & Ruigendijk, E. (Eds.). (2011). Production-comprehension asymmetries in child language. In *Studies on language acquisition* (Vol. 43, pp. 1–15). Walter de Gruyter & Co.
Williams, K. T. (2018). *Expressive Vocabulary Test* (3rd ed.). NCS Pearson.

Visual-Motor Coordination

Basic Definitions

Visual-motor coordination may be referred to by a variety of terms, including perceptual-motor integration and fine motor coordination. All the terms refer to an individual's capacity to carry out tasks that require smooth eye-hand coordination. More fundamentally, testing in this domain examines the accuracy of an individual's perception of stimuli and their related ability to appropriately manipulate objects in the environment.

Why Measure Visual-Motor Coordination?

Eye-hand coordination underlies an individual's ability to engage in a wide variety of daily living activities and academic tasks. School-based written language exercises and art projects, and home-based needs to open jar lids or unwrap small, hard candies are prime examples of tasks that depend on good visual-motor coordination. Thus, without good visual-motor coordination, many daily tasks can interfere significantly with optimal functioning.

Similarly to problems in other domains, youngsters' coordination difficulties can be interpreted by adults as evidence of laziness, lack of effort, or poor cooperation. For example, youth who have impaired perceptual-motor integration often refuse or sabotage fine motor tasks, calling forth frustration from parents, caregivers, and teachers. Such youngsters can seem as if they are dismissing demands made of them. In fact, often the youngsters are simply trying to avoid displaying what they consider incompetence. Due to fundamental, neurobehavioral determinants, youngsters with physical coordination problems often cannot successfully carry out

© Springer Nature Switzerland AG 2021
N. E. Moss, L. Moss-Racusin, *Practical Guide to Child and Adolescent Psychological Testing*, Best Practices in Child and Adolescent Behavioral Health Care, https://doi.org/10.1007/978-3-030-73515-9_9

even seemingly simple tasks. Their struggles are exacerbated when they are stressed by external demands, time limits, or disapproval.

Psychological assessment findings can shed light on visual-motor coordination difficulties and help to reveal any underlying, impaired fine motor skills. Furthermore, test findings can distinguish between problems with visual perception versus with motor output, as well as among problems that are part of more global impairments (e.g., Intellectual Disability or an Autism Spectrum Disorder).

Common Patterns of Difficulty

Many school-aged youngsters display trouble with completing graphomotor tasks required as part of their studies. Such trouble takes the form of an awkward pencil grasp, poor handwriting, and/or misaligned math problems, among other possibilities. Some youngsters display equal difficulty with fine motor tasks required to participate in everyday life. This difficulty may manifest as struggles to tie shoes or to button up a shirt.

How Do We Help?

Psychological test instruments are able to detect visual-motor problems, but they offer little intervention guidance. As with the speech and language domain of psychological testing, if basic psychological assessment findings indicate the presence of an impairment in visual-motor coordination, the youth should be referred for more specialized assessment (e.g., by a neurologist, physical therapist, or occupational therapist). In the primary care setting, providers may be in an excellent position to facilitate these referrals.

It is often quite helpful to request an occupational therapy evaluation. Occupational therapists have highly specialized knowledge regarding the motor coordination and motor planning skills needed to navigate successfully in both academic and daily life settings. Individuals trained in occupational therapy are experts in linking inborn perceptual and motor abilities with the most efficient way to accomplish designated tasks. Once an occupational therapy evaluation is completed, the relative utility of pursuing a full course of occupational therapy versus of making less formal adjustments in daily life routines can be determined.

An additional useful referral is for an assistive technology evaluation. Specialists in this area have cutting edge knowledge of the range of relevant technological assistance available to individuals in need of it. Careful, integrated analysis of all multidisciplinary assessment data, along with precise observations of a youngster's task-oriented behavior, allow the assistive technology specialist to recommend individualized strategies to enhance a youngster's functioning. For example, for a second grade student who becomes disruptive whenever written language

Table 1 Prominent instruments for assessing visual-motor coordination

Test name and publication date	Age range	Information provided by test
Beery-Buktenica Developmental Test of Visual-Motor Integration – Sixth Edition (BEERY VMI) 2010	2 years, 0 months – 99 years, 11 months	Visual and motor abilities integration

assignments are given in school, the assistive technology specialist might recommend a particular software program that provides an alternative, more comfortable way to complete the assignment by capitalizing on oral rather than visual-motor skills.

Prominent Instruments

Most test instruments in the visual-motor coordination domain rely on scoring of a person's paper-and-pencil ability to copy increasingly complex geometric forms. Drawn copies are scored for accuracy in shape, orientation, integration, and number. Alternate forms of instruments allow a psychologist to distinguish between problems that are primarily visual-perceptual, as opposed to those that mainly involve an individual's motor skills.

Among psychologists, the Beery-Buktenica Developmental Test of Visual-Motor Integration (BEERY VMI; Beery et al., 2010) is a popular instrument in the visual-motor coordination domain. Since the test examines an individual's competence at copying, tracing, and visually examining geometric forms of increasing complexity, it yields data regarding the accuracy of a youth's visual perception, proficiency with fine motor movements, and ability to integrate both visual input and motor output (Table 1).

Reference

Beery, K. E., Buktenica, N. A., & Beery, N. A. (2010). *Beery VMI: With supplemental developmental tests of visual perception and motor coordination and stepping stones age norms from birth to age six: Administration, scoring and teaching manual*. Pearson.

Memory

Basic Definitions

Memory testing involves assessment of a youth's retention, recall, and recognition of information. Several types of memory functions are relevant in a psychological assessment. These types vary by the kind of information to be remembered and the time span in which the information is recalled.

Verbal and visual material constitute the two main kinds of information that are of primary interest in psychological testing. The verbal domain involves orally conveyed, isolated information segments (e.g., single words), as well as broader narratives (e.g., a brief story). The visual domain involves exposure to pictorial information. Visual information can be in the form of abstract shapes of varying complexity or in the form of photographs or drawings of actual objects or people.

In regard to time span, immediate rote recall, short-term memory, long-term memory, and working memory are all important. Rote recall involves presentation of information segments followed immediately by a request for repetition of the information presented. Short-term and long-term memory refer to periods of information storage. To investigate these storage periods, assessment instruments often include presentation of information followed by varying delays before quizzing the individual on this information. Working memory involves the capacity to keep information in mind while carrying out an activity. For example, working memory is required when a teacher directs a student to complete an in-class assignment based on directions that are provided only once and that must be kept in mind.

© Springer Nature Switzerland AG 2021   63
N. E. Moss, L. Moss-Racusin, *Practical Guide to Child and Adolescent Psychological Testing*, Best Practices in Child and Adolescent Behavioral Health Care, https://doi.org/10.1007/978-3-030-73515-9_10

Why Measure Memory?

To provide adequate answers to many referral questions, it is essential to determine a youth's memory functioning (i.e., their ability to retain, recall, and recognize information). In many instances, without psychological assessment findings, it would be impossible to understand the interaction between memory operations and intellectual, academic, and behavioral challenges.

Once the nature of a youngster's memory functioning is well understood, a psychologist can offer guidance about how best to teach and interact with a youngster. Test instruments help indicate whether there is any difference in a youngster's memory efficiency in relation to information type or time span. If differences are noted, strategies should be designed to present information in the most manageable form and with proper assistance for required time periods. In this way, instruction is tailored to the youngster's strengths in order to maximize their capacity to remember important information.

It is important to note that memory test results are often impacted by a child or adolescent's attentional capacities. For memory operations to come into play, an individual must first be able to attend to information in their environment. More specifically, if a youngster has significant trouble with distractibility and/or sustained concentration, they have less opportunity to acquire information to be remembered. As a result, findings on tests of memory are often interpreted in the context of further findings on tests of attention and concentration.

Common Patterns of Difficulty

Impaired Rote Recall/Short-Term Memory

Nature of Difficulty Some psychological tests present novel information to an individual and progress quickly to examination of how much information is retained. This immediate examination yields findings related to rote recall, while examination that is carried out after a brief delay reflects short-term memory capacity. Individuals with true memory problems in either of these areas of functioning may give every indication of understanding information that is communicated to them, but then are unable to retain, recall, or recognize a sufficient amount of the information. In describing children and adolescents with this sort of problem, medical professionals, caregivers, and teachers often voice concerns such as, "I just said this. How can they not know?" or "We just reviewed this, and now it's as if they've never seen it!"

Problems in this area have several possible sources. As mentioned earlier, a memory problem may be rooted in attentional difficulties. That is, if an individual cannot attend to stimuli well enough for reliable initial input of information, then it will be impossible for the information to be stored in memory. Another possible source is intrusive anxiety that preempts focus on and absorption of information. Thirdly, rote recall and short-term memory problems may be one aspect of a major developmental disorder (e.g., Intellectual Disability or Autism Spectrum Disorder). Finally, such problems can be expressions of frank malfunctioning in memory operations.

How Do We Help? To improve rote recall and short-term memory, adults can assist children and adolescents by suggesting the following three strategies. First, youngsters should be alerted and readied to receive important information. Such an alert can be very simple. Often, the youngster just needs to be warned that critical information is about to be communicated, and then be encouraged to attend well.

Second, the youngster should be helped to create a method of repetition to anchor the information internally. This repetition can involve a verbal routine or a visualization process. To illustrate, a student can create an immediate, sing-song, internal repetition of communicated material in order to cement the material in their memory. They can also mentally "store" information in very familiar settings (e.g., pair each item in a list with the items of furniture in their bedroom).

Third, it is often productive to design mnemonic devices to supplement inadequate memory operations. These devices can and should be very concrete and mechanical. Many times, they involve associating information that needs to be remembered with tangible materials. As an illustration, a student faced with a challenging exam may decide to tie different colored strings on each of their fingertips, with each color representing a unique set of facts that would be covered on the exam.

It is very often true that children and adolescents themselves offer the best suggestions for memory improvement strategies to be adopted. Youngsters can make these suggestions once they fully understand the nature of their memory vulnerabilities and the rationale for helping themselves in this area. A youngster's creativity and willingness to implement strategies is often very encouraging.

Working Memory

Nature of Difficulty Trouble keeping essential information in mind while carrying out necessary tasks indicates a problem with working memory. For example, a student who forgets the criteria for a sorting task in the middle of the task likely has poor working memory. Working memory deficits are often associated with broader executive functioning problems and developmental disorders.

How Do We Help? Two main forms of assistance are useful for deficits in working memory. First, adults should teach children and adolescents cognitive self-awareness and self-regulation. The more a child or adolescent learns to monitor their own functioning, the better they can become at tasks requiring good working memory. Children and adolescents should be helped to schedule fixed intervals at which to stop and assess their current activity. Such checking reorients them to a task at hand and assists them in reinforcing recall of what they are supposed to be doing.

Second, technological aids are of significant value in addressing working memory problems. Technology aimed at relieving working memory impairments actually takes over some of the memory function. Video games used in classrooms that include periodic reminders of the games' rules are good examples of this method of helping with working memory problems. A wristwatch able to sound a quiet alarm at regular, pre-programmed intervals is another good example of how a technological aid can remind a youngster to review requirements of a task.

Deficits in Long-Term Memory

Nature of Difficulty Some individuals have an ability to acquire and retain information in the immediate and in the short-term, but struggle to retain that information for longer periods of time. Such memory problems can cause understandable frustration for affected children and adolescents, as well as for their parents, caregivers, teachers, and providers. For example, kind, determined efforts to explain an upcoming medical procedure to a young patient can appear to be successful, but then by the time the procedure is scheduled, the youngster has forgotten the explanation.

Sources of long-term memory problems are similar to the sources of immediate recall and short-term memory problems. Indeed, inattentiveness during initial exposure to information, intrusive anxiety and other comorbid disorders, and underlying deficits in brain function can all contribute to long-term memory problems.

How Do We Help? Proper nutrition and sleep are essential to good long-term memory functioning. Beyond these elements, to bolster long-term memory function, youngsters should have ample opportunities for repetition and practice of information. Adult guidance should be aimed at supporting youngsters in returning multiple times to the material that needs to be remembered. It is often most useful if practice and repetition sessions are separated by regular intervals. This separation allows for consolidation of information that can then be bolstered by additional exposure.

A second strategy for boosting long-term memory operation is to help a youngster identify cues that can trigger a body of knowledge. For example, a silly acronym can be associated with a set of facts that might otherwise be difficult to retrieve. Similar environments and states (e.g., sitting at a desk in a library) can also serve as recall cues.

   In addition to basic health, abundant repetition and practice, as well as cues, technological aids can also be useful in minimizing negative consequences of poor long-term memory functioning by serving storage and retrieval-of-information functions. For example, when a child or adolescent simply cannot retain particular information over time (e.g., all the foods to which they are allergic), a list saved in the notes section of their phone can reduce stress and provide essential guidance.

Table 1 Prominent instruments for assessing memory

Test name and publication date	Age range	Information provided by test
Wide Range Assessment of Memory and Learning – Second Edition (WRAML2) 2003	5 years – 90 years	Verbal memory Visual memory Attention/concentration Working memory Delayed memory Recognition

Prominent Instruments

The Wide Range Assessment of Memory and Learning (WRAML2; Sheslow & Adams, 2003) is a popular instrument in the assessment of memory. It examines all of the memory-related functions discussed above. Specifically, the WRAML2 (Sheslow & Adams, 2003) assesses both verbal and visual memory. Within each of these areas, subtests contrast an individual's competence with abstract versus concrete, meaningful information. For example, in the verbal memory subdomain, one subtest (Story Memory) presents coherent narratives, while the other (Verbal Learning) presents lists of isolated words. In the visual memory subdomain, one subtest (Design Memory) presents increasingly complex combinations of geometric forms, while another subtest (Picture Memory) presents drawings of everyday scenes.

Furthermore, the WRAML2 (Sheslow & Adams, 2003) assesses attention and concentration in relation to both orally presented, straightforward, isolated information segments (Number Letter) and to a more complex visual array requiring integration of visual input and kinesthetic output (Finger Windows). The WRAML2 (Sheslow & Adams, 2003) goes on to investigate working memory involving both words (Verbal Working Memory) and numbers and letters (Symbolic Working Memory). Finally, it evaluates the effects of time delays, as well as the benefits of providing recognition cues in both verbal and visual memory operations. Analysis of an individual's relative proficiency in all of these subdomains allows a psychologist to recommend intervention styles most likely to capitalize on an individual's strengths and thereby to promote the best retention of information (Table 1).

Reference

Sheslow, D., & Adams, W. (2003). *WRAML2: Wide Range Assessment of Memory and Learning.* Wide Range, Inc.

Attention and Concentration

Basic Definitions

Assessment in this domain examines a youngster's neurologically-based capacity to screen out distracting stimulation; focus on the most important information, activity, or communication in their immediate environment; and then sustain concentration on this information, activity, or communication for an optimal amount of time. Specific aspects of attentional functioning are also investigated. These include attention to auditory versus visual information, attention to simple segments of information versus complex information that requires more advanced mental manipulations, attention to fundamentally interesting versus more monotonous information, and the ability to maintain attention and concentration even in the face of interference from new information and task demands.

Why Measure Attention and Concentration?

Attentional functioning is an underpinning of all areas of behavior. To display one's intelligence accurately, learn successfully, participate comfortably in interpersonal interactions, and respond appropriately to directions, a child or adolescent must be able to reliably attend to and concentrate on input from the environment. If unable to attend and concentrate, all other domains of functioning are negatively impacted. The distracted individual, often feeling frustrated and ashamed, may resort to inappropriate behavioral strategies in an effort to camouflage or compensate for their inadequate attentional functioning. Others may underestimate the individual's true abilities due to the dampening effect of distractibility. Inaccurate judgments about the source of observable difficulty lead to incorrect interventions, and thereby make the problems worse.

© Springer Nature Switzerland AG 2021
N. E. Moss, L. Moss-Racusin, *Practical Guide to Child and Adolescent Psychological Testing*, Best Practices in Child and Adolescent Behavioral Health Care, https://doi.org/10.1007/978-3-030-73515-9_11

In contrast, if fundamental problems with marshaling attention and sustaining concentration are identified accurately through psychological testing, helpful interventions can be implemented. Affected individuals can be helped to bolster their self-esteem by understanding the inborn, rather than intentional, basis of their attentional problems. All those interacting with the distractible individual can gain assistance in factoring the attentional problems into more accurate appraisals of the individual. Effective treatment strategies, involving medication, counseling, and environmental structure, can be undertaken. In sum, then, assessment of attention and concentration in a youngster who is having difficulty is critically important in both developing an accurate formulation of the youngster's problems and in pointing the way toward useful interventions.

Common Patterns of Difficulty

Impaired Ability to Focus Attention

Nature of Difficulty On psychological testing, some youngsters manifest impairment in their capacity to zero in on a designated task, activity, or person. From the outset, they do not pay attention, instead attending haphazardly to many random stimuli. These stimuli can be internal sensations, preoccupations, or thoughts, as well as elements in the external environment such as sounds, behaviors of others, or objects at hand. This inability to focus attention may be accompanied by excessive physical activity (i.e., hyperactivity), but it may also occur in individuals whose outwardly observable physical activity level is entirely within normal limits.

As discussed earlier, the distractibility of a child or adolescent with this type of attentional difficulty may often be a source of frustration for adults, including primary care providers. Adults may misinterpret an inattentive youngster's behavior as willful ignoring of adult input. In fact, the youngster may have variable awareness of their poor attentional functioning. An otherwise easy-going, pleasant child or adolescent may not realize in the moment that their attention fluctuates in disruptive ways. There is often a painful mismatch between adult impatience with what seems to be obvious disregard for expectations and a youth's amiable outlook. In such situations, children and adolescents can feel hurt or resentful in response to adult disapproval. Moreover, the youngster's self-esteem often suffers.

Youngsters who have trouble focusing their attention also often encounter peer relationship problems. It is difficult for a child or adolescent with compromised attention to participate fully and appropriately in social activities. Peers may misinterpret the inattentiveness of a distractible youngster as indicating that the youngster simply does not like them, and respond accordingly. Indeed, children and adolescents often struggle to correctly identify the actual source of an interpersonal problem and may personalize it (Muris & Field, 2008). Additionally, peers may experience highly distractible behavior as unsettling. In response to their discomfort, these peers might self-protectively pull away from the youngster with poor attentional functioning. The resulting social isolation can be painful. Older and/or self-aware youngsters may see all too clearly the ways in which their poor attentional functioning blocks academic, vocational, and social success. Such youngsters often wrestle with disappointing comparisons between the life that they wish for and the life that they experience.

Inadequate Concentration

Nature of Difficulty In some cases, psychological test findings indicate that an individual can manage to focus their initial attention but cannot sustain their concentration. Such a youngster would, for example, respond well to a teacher's direction regarding getting out a required workbook, and might even listen closely enough to grasp the teacher's explanation about how to tackle an assignment, but then be found daydreaming or doing something entirely unrelated instead of following through with independent effort. Both internal and external stimuli can interfere with maintenance of concentration, and this interference is almost always outside the youngster's awareness. All of the interpersonal and self-esteem issues described above in relation to impairment of attention are also relevant to individuals with impairment of concentration.

Inappropriate Regulation of Attention

Nature of Difficulty For some individuals, the problem is not with initial focus or sustained concentration but rather with the regulation of attentional functioning. Children and adolescents in this group are often described as becoming completely lost in an object or activity of high interest. Such youngsters can hyper-focus so extremely on high interest areas that they are unaware of happenings in their immediate environment. Without interruption, they might remain in this state for extended periods of time. When interruptions inevitably occur, these youth may have great difficulty transitioning successfully to another activity. Again, as with the individuals with other attentional impairments, youngsters who cannot regulate their attentional functioning are likely to experience productivity, self-esteem, and interpersonal challenges.

How Do We Help?

Children and adolescents in all three of these groups can be helped by individualized assistance plans that draw from the same set of strategies. In the interest of limiting the intrusiveness of interventions and of minimizing vulnerability to unwanted health impacts, the first two strategies should always be tried first. Often, they will be successful. If they are not, the third strategy should be provided as a source of much-needed relief for more severely affected youngsters.

Psychoeducation Even more than is true for many other disorders, psychoeducation is the first critical component of assisting youngsters with compromised attention. These youngsters typically have a history of feeling badly about themselves when they are unable to respond adequately to requests or demands for their steady, appropriate attention, and they often blame themselves as much as others do. They may also mask their insecurity and self-blame with overtly inappropriate, angry behavior. To access their energy and motivation to improve, youngsters with poor attentional functioning need to be taught that their attentional problems are rooted in their nervous systems, not manifesting their supposed inferiority. They need to be helped to lessen their self-blame. They are then likely to be able to approach their attentional difficulties with a much more adaptive, problem-solving attitude.

Environmental Interventions Second, a large number of environmental interventions can be implemented to enhance a youngster's attentional functioning. Overall, these environmental interventions should be aimed at providing the most structured environment possible for the youth. They can be adapted to home, school, medical, and other environments in which the youngster needs to operate. The specific interventions that will be most successful will vary according to each individual's strengths and weaknesses. Adults should experiment, incorporating the youngster's input, in order to design and then refine the most effective interventions. However, generally useful environmental interventions include the following.

Explicit Expectations There should be a clear set of behavioral and task-oriented expectations for a child or adolescent to meet. Adults should ensure that the expectations are in keeping with the youngster's developmental status and capacities. The child or adolescent should be clearly informed about all of the relevant expectations. Any necessary explanations to make it possible for the youngster to succeed should be provided. The youngster's input should be incorporated into the set of expectations, as appropriate. For cases in which implementation of explicit expectations proves impossible, a behavior management plan (discussed further in the Behavioral Functioning chapter) should be designed.

Predictable Schedule Youngsters with compromised attentional capabilities do best with a reliable, predictable schedule. At home, in school, and in other environments where a youngster spends appreciable amounts of time, the order and duration of events and activities should be laid out clearly. Particularly for younger children, a visual representation of the schedule is often very helpful as a tangible anchor point. Every effort should be made to avoid deviations from that schedule, even if those deviations appear to be pleasant and enjoyable surprises. The disorganization that results from disrupting the schedule usually overshadows any brief enjoyment that might result.

Brief Instructions Directions should be short and precise in order to maximize the possibility that the distractible youngster will listen to all of them. Directions should include guidance about what the youngster should do if they forget previously delivered instructions. For example, if a youngster forgets their chores, they should have been informed to consult the list of their chores hanging on the refrigerator.

Segmented Efforts When a youngster with concentration problems is expected to carry out sustained effort (e.g. to write a term paper or to clean their bedroom), it is useful to divide the work into a series of segments. As an example, one section of the term paper could be written at a time, and one quadrant of the bedroom could be cleaned at a time. Tackling individual segments of a task is less daunting and more achievable than taking on the whole task at once. Furthermore, completing each segment offers a much-needed sense of accomplishment, which is reinforcing.

Frequent Breaks To facilitate success for distractible youngsters, they should be encouraged to take frequent breaks when engaging in effortful work. Breaks may be quite short; even a few minutes can help an individual to rouse their attention and reinforce their focus. They should not exceed approximately fifteen minutes. For young children, breaks should be regularly scheduled based on adult appraisal of needs. For older children and adolescents with enough self-awareness, breaks can be taken at their own discretion, and they can be taught to signal a relevant adult that a break is needed. Acceptable behavior and location during breaks should be specified in advance. Ideally, youngsters will spend their breaks doing a preferred activity that is acceptable within the particular environment. For some youngsters, a physical activity to "get the wiggles out" may be most effective.

Reduced Workload Also for individuals with pronounced trouble sustaining concentration, it is helpful to evaluate the size of the workload assigned to them. Assignments should be examined in order to determine exactly what knowledge the student is expected to demonstrate through it. In many cases, the student can provide an adequate demonstration of that knowledge with a briefer assignment. To illustrate, if a page of math homework contains 20 problems, a student with impaired concentration could do all of the odd-numbered problems. Likely, there would be a minimal loss of math practice and development, but an appreciable benefit for the student's successful work completion.

Controlled External Distractions To support individuals with attentional problems, careful appraisal is required to determine whether background noise and activity either promotes or hinders purposeful effort. For some distractible youngsters, steady, repetitive sound in their environment (e.g., music at low volume or a murmured family conversation) helps them to focus. For others, any external stimulation is so distracting that it prevents all meaningful work. For these latter individuals, work areas should have a minimum of extraneous materials, sights, and sounds. In a classroom, portable dividers can be used to create relatively secluded study areas containing only materials essential for task completion. In the home, electronic diversions and tempting family activities can be deferred until necessary tasks are finished.

Proximity Management   Youngsters with attentional difficulties often require more than a typical amount of guidance from adults in their environment. For each setting in which an affected youngster is expected to work productively, nearness to an adult authority should be considered. Most often, it is best for a distractible child or adolescent to have the easiest possible access to the adult. Such close contact is typically very reassuring and facilitates obtaining information and answers to questions as they arise. In a classroom, proximity can be satisfied by offering seating close to teachers. In other environments, the exact best location is variable but should always provide close proximity to a needed adult.

Close Supervision   Even when all of the aforementioned environmental interventions are provided, a youngster with an attentional difficulty may still struggle significantly to stay on task. There is no substitute for close supervision by teachers, parents, and caregivers. This supervision should be aimed at helping the youngster to resist both external and internal distractions and to redirect to meaningful work when lapses in attention and concentration do occur. Every effort should be made to keep this close supervision free of a punitive tone, as well as appropriately reinforcing when good performance occurs.

Medication   For a great many youngsters with compromised attention and concentration, the strategies of psychoeducation and environmental interventions are sufficient to achieve marked improvement. However, there are individuals with more extreme difficulties for whom psychoeducation and environmental interventions alone do not provide sufficient relief. These individuals should receive medical consultation to explore the potential usefulness of medication support. Primary care providers are well-suited to provide this consultation and to prescribe, as appropriate, for children and adolescents with clear-cut attentional problems. For those youngsters who have more complex diagnostic presentations that include comorbid mental health disorders, support from professionals trained in psychiatric medication is generally more prudent.

Often, parents and caregivers are reluctant to pursue medication to treat attentional problems in children and adolescents. Concerns include penalizing "just being a kid," causing bodily harm, promoting drug dependence, transforming basic personality, undermining self-reliance and self-discipline. Adults are right to be cautious and careful in all decisions concerning the youngsters for whom they are responsible. No decision is absolutely risk-free. However, for severe attentional problems, medication can be enormously helpful.

To address parent and caregiver reluctance to use medication, it can first be helpful to provide ample information about the medication's function and likely effects. The adults should be allowed to ask any relevant questions. Reassurance should be offered truthfully (i.e., that most of the typical medications used to treat attentional problems are relatively low risk in relation to all of the productivity, self-esteem, and interpersonal concerns listed above (Cortese et al., 2018; Smith et al., 2000)). A methodical approach, with regular observation and monitoring, should be proposed for beginning medication.

Most importantly, it is helpful to discuss with parents and caregivers the high cost of withholding medication from some children and adolescents. For youngsters whose daily functioning is severely hampered by their inabilities to focus appropriately and to concentrate continuously, doing without medication can force them into persistent failure and unhappiness in multiple important life domains. Youngsters who receive much-needed medication are often the most eloquent in attesting to its academic and social benefits; it is common to hear them comment, "I never knew I could feel this way," or "Is this how most people feel all the time?" A cautious but open-minded attitude toward the medical treatment of attentional problems is reasonable and should be encouraged.

Prominent Instruments

Test instruments used to measure attention and concentration are divided between checklist reports of daily functioning in everyday settings and direct measures administered in the assessment setting. Prime examples of checklist reports include the Conners (Conners 3; Conners, 2008) and the Barkley Adult ADHD Rating Scale (BAARS-IV; Barkley, 2011). Respondents who know the youngster well, along with the youngster themselves (if old and capable enough to participate), review lists of behavioral descriptions related to attentional functioning. The respondent then uses a numerical scale to indicate how often the designated behavior occurs. Scoring systems then allow for determination of an individual's attentional competence.

NEPSY-II (Korkman et al., 2007) subtests such as Auditory Attention and Response Set, along with the computerized Conners' Continuous Performance Test (Conners CPT 3; Conners, 2014), are prominent examples of direct measures of attention and concentration. With each of these instruments, the individual being tested is presented with lengthy, inherently uninteresting segments of information. The individual is instructed to perform a very simple, rote task (e.g., point to a picture on paper or respond to a computer image) under differing sets of instructions. Immediate rote attention, continuous vigilance and concentration, containment of impulsivity, disregard for competing distractions in the environment, and maintenance of energy for task compliance are all required to do well on these tests.

To best understand the youth being tested, it is particularly important to compare and contrast findings regarding attention and concentration in daily life versus in the assessment setting. Some individuals are quite competent at marshaling their attention and sustaining their concentration in calm, quiet settings, where there is relatively little environmental interference. These same individuals may simply be

Table 1 Prominent instruments for assessing attention and concentration

Test name and publication date	Age range	Information provided by test
Conners 3rd Edition (Conners 3) 2008	6 years – 18 years for teacher and parent rating scales 8 years – 18 years for self-report	Hyperactivity/impulsivity Executive functioning Learning problems Aggression Peer relations Family relations Inattention
Barkley Adult ADHD Rating Scale-IV (BAARS-IV) 2011	18 years – 89 years	Current ADHD symptoms Recollections of childhood symptoms
NEPSY – Second Edition (NEPSY-II) 2007	3 years – 16 years	Executive function and attention Language Memory and learning Sensorimotor Visuospatial processing Social perception
Conners' Continuous Performance Test 3rd Edition (Conners CPT 3) 2014	8+ years	Inattentiveness Impulsivity Sustained attention Vigilance

unable to maintain good attentional functioning in settings with more activity, people, and objects, though. Other individuals are energized by a great deal of seemingly distracting environmental input but are unable to display good attentional functioning in a quieter, more secluded setting. Still other individuals display consistent attentional functioning regardless of setting. Psychological test results can document an individual's pattern of attentional performance across settings and thereby identify the environmental circumstances under which they can manifest their best capacities (Table 1).

References

Barkley, R. A. (2011). *BAARS-IV: Barkley Adult ADHD Rating Scale*. Guilford Press.

Conners, C. K. (2008). *Conners' Rating Scales*. Multi-Health Systems.

Conners, C. K. (2014). *Conners' Continuous Performance Test, (3rd ed.; Conners CPT 3) & Conners' Continuous Auditory Test of Attention (Conners CATA): Technical manual*. Multi-Health Systems.

Cortese, S., Adamo, N., Del Giovane, C., Mohr-Jensen, C., Hayes, A. J., Carucci, S., Atkinson, L. Z., Tessari, L., Banaschewski, T., Coghill, D., Hollis, C., Simonoff, E., Zuddas, A., Barbui, C., Purgato, M., Steinhausen, H.-C., Shokraneh, F., Xia, J., & Cipriani, A. (2018). Comparative efficacy and tolerability of medications for Attention-Deficit Hyperactivity Disorder in children, adolescents, and adults: A systematic review and network meta-analysis. *The Lancet Psychiatry, 5*(9), 727–738. https://doi.org/10.1016/S2215-0366(18)30269-4

Smith, B. H., Waschbusch, D. A., Willoughby, M. T., & Evans, S. (2000). The efficacy, safety, and practicality of treatments for adolescents with Attention-Deficit/Hyperactivity Disorder (ADHD). *Clinical Child and Family Psychology Review, 3*, 243–267. https://doi.org/10.102 3/A:1026477121224

Korkman, M., Kirk, U., & Kemp, S. (2007). *NEPSY-II* (2nd ed.). Psychological Corporation.

Muris, P., & Field, A. P. (2008). Distorted cognition and pathological anxiety in children and adolescents. *Cognition and Emotion, 22*(3), 395–421. https://doi.org/10.1080/02699930701843450

Executive Functioning

Basic Definitions

Executive functioning in relation to psychological functioning and assessment refers to higher order mental organization, self-regulation, and the capacity to engage in efficient, planful action. Goal-setting, time management, marshaling resources, making mid-course corrections, and keeping sight of the overall relevant situation are all important aspects of executive functioning. More particularly, executive functioning can be understood in three related domains, explicated below.

Emotional Regulation

This sphere of executive functioning involves the ability to manage and control feelings well enough to prevent them from disrupting appropriate behavior and task accomplishment. Being able to manage transitions between activities without becoming unduly frustrated or upset is a skill characteristic of a youngster with good emotional executive functioning.

Behavioral Regulation

This sphere of executive functioning refers to keeping observable behaviors sufficiently in check to allow for meaningful activity. Specifically, a youngster needs to be able to refrain from engaging in behaviors unrelated or in opposition to the task at hand. Just as importantly, a youngster needs to be able to monitor their own behavior to guarantee that they continue to be appropriately goal-directed.

© Springer Nature Switzerland AG 2021

N. E. Moss, L. Moss-Racusin, *Practical Guide to Child and Adolescent Psychological Testing*, Best Practices in Child and Adolescent Behavioral Health Care, https://doi.org/10.1007/978-3-030-73515-9_12

Cognitive Regulation

This sphere of executive functioning pertains to the mental efforts required to remain on task. These efforts include formulating and implementing a plan for task initiation, keeping information in mind while carrying out related tasks, planning and organizing effective action, accurately monitoring progress toward task completion, and organizing necessary materials.

Why Measure Executive Functioning?

Just as a corporation needs a competent Chief Executive Officer to guide and manage all corporate activities, so too does an individual require solid, steady executive functioning to navigate responsibly through daily life. Good executive functioning helps children and adolescents meet such common demands as following classroom routines, demonstrating good study habits, completing homework in a timely fashion, keeping track of belongings, and finishing chores. Executive functioning is thus one of many components that contribute to overall wellbeing and success.

Impaired executive functioning is often an aspect of various disorders found in childhood and adolescence. Attention-Deficit/Hyperactivity Disorder and Autism Spectrum Disorder are two prominent examples of disorders that typically include compromised executive functioning as part of their presentation. It is possible, though, to find problematic executive functioning as a youngster's singular difficulty or as a facet of other childhood or adolescent disorders. Since executive functioning has such powerful implications for an individual's capacity to be successful, accurate assessment of this area of a youngster's functioning is essential.

Common Patterns of Difficulty

Impaired Emotional Regulation

Nature of Difficulty To meet designated responsibilities and carry out necessary functions, an individual needs to be able to manage their levels of emotional arousal and expression. Without good regulation of emotional experience, feelings interfere too much in task accomplishment. Therefore, abrupt shifts between different feelings and extreme, intrusive fluctuations in the intensity of emotional experience characterize poor emotional regulation. Examples of youngsters with poor emotional regulation include a student whose anger is so explosive it leads to ripping up a challenging homework assignment, and a patient whose unchecked anxiety stops them from speaking straightforwardly to their primary care provider about a persistent stomachache.

Excessive distress in the face of real or perceived failure on a task is a common manifestation of impaired emotional regulation among children and adolescents.

Rather than fairly assessing the results of their efforts, youngsters with impaired emotional executive functioning often interpret any outcome short of perfection as a terrible failure. They then make a quick leap to negative self-evaluation. Further distress over this assault on their self-esteem adds an additional obstacle to reapplying themselves to the task at hand.

How Do We Help? For many years, an individual's executive functioning was viewed as relatively fixed and permanent. Clinicians and educators believed that little could be done to impact executive functioning level. Over time, though, it has become clear that concrete, educational strategies can be very helpful in improving executive functioning (e.g., Gagne & Nwadinobi, 2018).

The primary way to help with impaired emotional regulation is to teach the affected youngster two main skills. First, the youngster needs assistance in recognizing the emotions they are feeling. While it may seem obvious to outside observers, the child or adolescent is often so overwhelmed by an emotional experience that they cannot think clearly about what they are feeling. It is helpful to teach them to notice signals, such as in their bodily expressions (e.g., clenched fists), which they can link with particular emotions. Then, they can be helped to better understand the sources and effects of their emotions.

Second, youngsters should be taught self-soothing strategies that can help them return to a more tolerable emotional level. There are many forms of such strategies from which to choose. Mindfulness meditative practices and breathing techniques can be immensely helpful; myriad applications and programs with these practices and techniques are available on computers and phones. For some youngsters, designing even the simplest individualized self-soothing strategy can be extremely effective. For example, a student with a mild Intellectual Disability who is easily riled up whenever they do not understand an instruction or comment from a teacher can be taught and encouraged to very slowly count their fingers in these instances. The time and concentration that such a counting task demands will likely deflate irritation and allow the student to proceed more appropriately.

To be complete, the teaching of self-soothing strategies should include explicit suggestions about when, where, and for how long to carry out a self-regulatory practice. Without this explicit instruction, youngsters with poor emotional regulation could easily compound their problems by attempting to use self-soothing strategies inappropriately. For example, a youngster might attempt a self-soothing strategy once for two seconds, declare it has not cured their problem, and then panic that they are beyond help.

Impaired Behavioral Regulation

Nature of Difficulty Individuals with problems with behavioral regulation typically engage either in unnecessary activities that they consider preparatory for a designated task or in activities that allow them to withdraw from challenges that they cannot manage. To illustrate, when struggling to write a term paper, an anxious and depressed high school student may spend a great deal of time arranging the objects on their desk. Then, even though the paper is already outlined, they review all of their notes and rewrite a list of the main points that they wish to make in the paper. For youngsters of all ages, video games often figure prominently in manifestations of poor behavioral regulation. A behaviorally dysregulated youngster often spends countless hours playing games on screens rather than attending to designated responsibilities.

How Do We Help? It is often useful to begin efforts to help youngsters with impaired behavioral regulation by increasing their internally-based strategies. Such strategies reinforce independence, allowing the youngster to feel justifiably proud and self-reliant. Specifically, internally-based strategies should be directed at improving the youth's self-monitoring. One example of a strategy to enhance self-monitoring is check points, which can be initiated, for instance, by programmed alerts on a phone. When an alert sounds, or any type of marker event occurs, a youngster can be taught to stop what they are doing and evaluate the appropriateness of their actions. If on task, the child or adolescent can continue productively. If off task, they can use this check point as a reminder to return to more appropriate activity.

For some youngsters, self-monitoring is simply too difficult. They cannot successfully regulate their behavioral executive functioning without direct assistance from others. For these youngsters, it is often best to design and implement a detailed, individualized behavior management plan (described in detail in the Behavioral Functioning chapter) that targets problem-solving and task accomplishment. A behavior management plan for executive functioning should include designation of the relevant task, specification of behaviors consistent with task accomplishment and extraneous to it, design of a timeline leading to accomplishment, inclusion of check-ins with an appropriate adult to ensure steady progress, and agreement about acceptable rewards and consequences dependent on performance. Sometimes, youngsters derive enough benefit from such a behavior management plan that they are then able to move forward toward more independent self-monitoring.

Impaired Cognitive Regulation

Nature of Difficulty Children and adolescents who have difficulty with cognitive regulation struggle to keep their minds operating in an orderly manner. Difficulty in this domain is characterized by marked disorganization in thoughts, actions, and use of time and materials. Often, despite the best of intentions, individuals with impaired cognitive regulation may, for example, begin one task, shift abruptly to thinking about another, realize that they do not have the necessary supplies to finish either task, head off to get those supplies but come back with only some of what they need, only to return to the first task in exhaustion. In a fundamental sense, they cannot control the efficiency of their thought processes.

How Do We Help? Organizing a highly structured procedure to follow is typically very effective for helping a youth with impaired cognitive regulation. The procedure should specify the starting point of a task and its end goal. A reasonable work space should be arranged. All needed supplies should be listed and obtained. The task should be divided into manageable portions. The duration of time required for each portion should be estimated. The youth should then be taught to use this procedure guide as the foundation for their present efforts, as well as for future task-planning and completion. They should check back with their procedure outline in order to assess progress and determine next steps.

As discussed above in regard to poor behavioral self-regulation, some children and adolescents with executive functioning problems cannot monitor their own efforts well enough to follow even a well-designed procedure. Usually, poor self-monitoring is the source of inability to adhere to an agreed upon procedure. When this is true, it is often best to implement the steps outlined earlier in regard to teaching better self-monitoring.

Prominent Instruments

Like measures of attentional functioning, measures of executive functioning distinguish between naturalistic behavior in everyday settings and behavior in structured test settings. The Second Edition of the Behavior Rating Inventory of Executive Function (BRIEF2; Gioia et al., 2015) and the Adult Version of the Behavior Rating Inventory of Executive Function (BRIEF-A; Roth et al., 2005) focus on executive functioning in typical, day-to-day situations. All forms of this instrument require either a respondent who is very familiar with the individual being tested or the individual themselves to complete a comprehensive checklist. The checklist items all pertain to possible real life manifestations of executive functioning problems. Analysis of the findings indicates the extent to which an individual's executive functioning is impaired. Measures such as some of the NEPSY-II (Korkman et al., 2007) subtests are useful in directly assessing an individual's executive functioning in the test setting. To illustrate, the Animal Sorting subtest yields information about an individual's ability to conceptualize and think flexibly. The Clock subtest measures planning capacity. The Inhibition subtest assesses an individual's ability to be productive under specific and changing constraints.

Integration of the findings on different types of measures is most useful. Some individuals have minimal executive functioning skill across settings. Others display their best executive functioning in a quiet, supportive, structured setting. Other individuals do best in a livelier, naturalistic setting. Still others can display good executive functioning under all conditions. Intervention-planning should be geared toward whatever profile an individual displays (Table 1).

Table 1 Prominent instruments for assessing executive functioning

Test name and publication date	Age range	Information provided by test
Behavior Rating Inventory of Executive Function, Second Edition (BRIEF2) 2015	5 years – 18 years	Behavioral regulation: Inhibit Self-monitor
		Emotional regulation: Shift Emotional control
		Cognitive regulation: Initiate Task completion Working memory Plan/organize Task-monitor Organization of materials
Behavior Rating Inventory of Executive Function – Adult Version (BRIEF-A) 2005	18 years – 90 years	Behavioral regulation: Inhibit Shift Emotional control Self-monitor Metacognition: Initiate Working memory Plan/organize Task monitor Organization of materials
NEPSY – Second Edition (NEPSY-II) 2007	3 years – 16 years	Executive function and attention Language Memory and learning Sensorimotor Visuospatial processing Social perception

References

Gagne, J. R., & Nwadinobi, O. K. (2018). Self-control interventions that benefit executive functioning and academic outcomes in early and middle childhood. *Early Education and Development, 29*(7), 971–987. https://doi.org/10.1080/10409289.2018.1496721

Gioia, G. A., Isquith, P. K., Guy, S. C., & Kenworthy, L. (2015). *BRIEF2: Behavior Rating Inventory of Executive Function* (2nd ed.). Psychological Assessment Resources.

Korkman, M., Kirk, U., & Kemp, S. (2007). *NEPSY-II* (2nd ed.). Psychological Corporation.

Roth, R. M., Isquith, P. K., & Gioia, G. A. (2005). *BRIEF-A: Behavior Rating Inventory of Executive Function, Adult Version*. Psychological Assessment Resources.

Academic Achievement

Basic Definitions

Academic achievement refers to the level of scholastic accomplishment reached by a child or adolescent. Although they are never completely separate from one another, it is critically important to differentiate learning levels from fundamental intelligence. While fundamental intelligence is the intellectual capacity with which each individual is born, scholastic accomplishment represents the extent to which an individual has been able to respond to instruction (i.e., to use their inborn intelligence to process information and thereby learn). Individuals are most comfortable when their academic achievement levels are equivalent to their basic intelligence.

Why Measure Academic Achievement?

Measurement of academic achievement is frequently included in a psychological test battery. Most often, such testing is included to understand and address a youngster's reported school-based difficulties. As noted earlier in regard to common reasons for pursuing psychological testing, when a child or adolescent is struggling with scholastic accomplishments in an adequate instructional setting, it is necessary to determine whether those struggles reflect learning problems or interference from problems of another sort (e.g., emotional or behavioral difficulties). Academic achievement test results are central in making such a determination. Test findings reveal the roots of difficulty acquiring academic knowledge at the normative rate and level. When there is formal difficulty with the learning process itself, a youngster is understood to have a Learning Disorder. With information from academic achievement testing, appropriate interventions, such as alternate instructional

© Springer Nature Switzerland AG 2021   85
N. E. Moss, L. Moss-Racusin, *Practical Guide to Child and Adolescent Psychological Testing*, Best Practices in Child and Adolescent Behavioral Health Care, https://doi.org/10.1007/978-3-030-73515-9_13

methods, individualized opportunities for displaying knowledge, changes in school setting, and other environmental modifications, can be pursued.

Common Patterns of Difficulty

Learning Disorder

Nature of Difficulty When a youngster's academic achievement skills surpass their measured intelligence by a significant margin, they should be understood as an overachiever. In contrast, when a youngster's academic achievement levels are significantly lower than their measured intelligence despite adequate instruction, they should be understood as having a Learning Disorder.

A note about approaches to diagnosing Learning Disorders is helpful here. Historically, Learning Disorders were identified using the "discrepancy model." In this model, a discrepancy of a designated size (i.e., 22 points) between better intelligence and weaker academic achievement was interpreted to mean that a youngster was unable to process certain types of information at a level predicted by their intellectual ability. This inability was believed to indicate that the individual had a Learning Disorder.

For a number of theoretical and practical reasons, the discrepancy model came under a great deal of criticism (Restori et al., 2009). In its place, educators chose to base identification of Learning Disorders on the "response to instruction model." In this model, youngsters are identified through academic achievement testing as having an inadequate response to appropriate instruction. Specified levels of additional instruction are then provided to attempt to improve a youngster's learning. If inadequate scholastic accomplishment persists despite multiple levels of instruction, a Learning Disorder is diagnosed. It is important to emphasize that this diagnosis is not made firmly until a youngster is old enough to have received a designated amount of instruction, and until initial attempts to close the achievement gap have failed. As a result, premature diagnoses are avoided, and attention stays focused on the quality of instruction delivered.

Learning Disorders are identified in the basic building-block academic subjects (i.e., reading, math, and written language). In reading, Learning Disorders can impact grasp of letter-sound relationships, more complex aspects of phonetic analysis and word decoding, visual tracking of the printed word, comprehension of the meaning of material that is read, and/or a combination of these elements. Reading Learning Disorders are often quite noticeable in classroom and family settings, and they can cause concern and embarrassment. They also interfere with achievement across subject areas as youngsters move upward in grade level, since with each succeeding grade level, it becomes more important for students to read in order to acquire information. Thus, a Learning Disorder in reading can slow progress even in academic areas that might otherwise be successful for a child or adolescent.

In math, Learning Disorders may manifest primarily as difficulty with computations. Such difficulty is often exacerbated by visual-motor struggles that interfere with proper alignment of math problems. Learning Disorders in math can also manifest as difficulty with word problems. Since word problems are presented in written form, any reading deficits can magnify struggles with math performance. In addition, some youngsters' Learning Disorders in math relate mainly to the speed at which they can do academic work. Slow mental processing interferes with elementary math operations (i.e., addition, subtraction, multiplication, and division), which need to become automatic for a student to progress to more complex math.

Finally, Learning Disorders in written language pertain to a youngster's skill at translating thoughts and spoken language into written form. A substantial number of youngsters can think about and discuss academic topics in a very competent manner, but struggle greatly to translate those thoughts and discussions into written form. They are blocked at the level of formulating appropriate language for the page or computer screen. Other youngsters throw themselves into writing with enthusiasm, but display numerous errors with spelling, punctuation, word choice, grammar, and sentence structure. If a child or adolescent has a written language Learning Disorder, these errors persist despite numerous corrections.

How Do We Help? Any attempt to ameliorate academic struggles must begin with verification of the nature and quality of the instruction that a youth has received. Psychologists who provide formal assessments are well trained to assist with such verification. Some school settings may be so limited by socioeconomic inequalities or overwhelmed by behavior problems that delivery of the core curriculum suffers greatly. Other schools that appear to be operating with every possible advantage may choose unique instructional timetables that defer emphasis on particular academic skills until higher than usual grade levels. If investigation reveals that a youngster's academic lags are associated with a demonstrable lack of instruction, the lack should be addressed before any Learning Disorder diagnosis is made. If, however, the youngster has had appropriate opportunity to master scholastic information but has not done so in a timely manner, a Learning Disorder diagnosis should be made.

Once an accurate Learning Disorder diagnosis has been made, the next helpful step is to offer relief if youngsters feel distressed about their academic struggles. While it is important to be honest and acknowledge that the Learning Disorder is a permanent fixture of their lives, youngsters should be reassured in the clearest terms that their impairments reflect nothing more than underlying, inherited features of their information-processing style. It can be difficult for many youngsters to believe and to internalize this reassurance. Instead, they may engage in negative self-evaluations, believing themselves to have caused their scholastic problems somehow. Since they can virtually never identify any such actions, they are typically left bewildered and dismayed.

Youngsters may also attribute their Learning Disorders to imagined fundamental aspects of their character or capacities, such as laziness or deficient intelligence. Unfortunately, criticism from poorly informed adults or mockery from peers may contribute to this erroneous belief. Believing themselves fundamentally flawed, youth may not pursue supports they deserve and from which they could benefit. Their dismay then only increases if even redoubled scholastic effort inevitably fails to eliminate the manifestations of the Learning Disorder.

Some young people may also associate their Learning Disorder with misbehavior. These children and adolescents develop a view of themselves as inherently bad. While it is often true that students with Learning Disorders exhibit disruptive behaviors, the behavioral disturbances cannot cause a Learning Disorder. It is much likelier that the inappropriate behavior represents a frustrated response to academic struggles or a wish to deflect attention away from them. Sadly, many youngsters can tolerate behavioral punishment more easily than recognition of fundamental limitations.

Again, it is essential to provide every possible reassurance against these manifestations of self-blame and self-criticism for a Learning Disorder. Furthermore, youngsters should be informed that there are specialized teaching strategies that can be utilized to enhance their learning. They should be told that they are legally entitled to a special education program that addresses their needs. (Please find additional information about the special education process in the Types of Psychological Assessments and the School Psychoeducational Assessment Process chapters.) Special education should be explained broadly to youngsters as a way for them to take in information and demonstrate knowledge that bypasses their mental processing limitations. A summary of some special education practices commonly used to address Learning Disorders is included here.

Use of technology can be significantly helpful. Such technology includes devices that present reading materials in adjusted formats and pair written words to be read with spoken words. Increasingly sophisticated calculators and computer programs take over basic arithmetic and higher math functions, allowing youngsters to concentrate on conceptual understanding. Additionally, a wide range of dictation software can substitute for traditional writing.

Certain special education approaches are most appropriate for specific types of Learning Disorders. To address Learning Disorders in reading, consultation with reading specialists should be obtained in order to choose the most appropriate curriculum materials. Beyond the curriculum, youngsters should also be offered audio recordings and video depictions of essential material. In this way, they can learn without having to rely upon their poor reading skills.

For Learning Disorders in math, concrete materials and manipulatives can be very helpful. At younger ages especially, using such tangible objects can promote learning better than numbers on a page or a screen. At all ages, using visualization can be useful. To illustrate, a student can imagine, or even draw, two groups of three oranges each and count the total number of fruits, rather than try to directly memorize that three times two equals six. Additionally, use of specially lined paper (e.g., graph paper) can help greatly when visual-motor difficulties are contributing to trouble solving math problems.

In regard to written language Learning Disorders, the key is to use alternate forms of displaying knowledge about scholastic material. Oral reports, debates, original songs, and myriad types of artistic rendering are just some of the ways that children and adolescents who struggle with writing can work around their limitations and take pride in the knowledge that they have acquired.

For some youths, additional personalized tutorial assistance beyond formal special education is also helpful. When resources are available to obtain this assistance, it can provide more instruction, practice, and familiarity with scholastic material, all of which can ultimately boost a youngster's self-confidence. To maximize the benefits of tutorial assistance, close coordination is essential between both the tutor's and the classroom instructor's curriculum materials and didactic methods. Without such coordination, a youngster is at risk for being caught between competing instructional approaches.

Unlike those of the mid-twentieth century, many current special education services are embedded in mainstream settings, although some one-to-one and small group services do also occur (Rotatori et al., 2011). Embedded service provision tends to enhance generalization of skills and to minimize students' feelings of isolation and embarrassment (Rakap & Parlak-Rakap, 2011). There are some cases where special education in the local school district proves insufficient, though. In these cases, placement is warranted in a specialized school designed specifically for youngsters with Learning Disorders. The expert staff at such schools can often help their students make notable academic progress. However, in addition to being quite expensive, out-placement can disrupt a youngster's relationships with their peers and community, as well as amplify their self-perception as someone apart from the mainstream. Great care should be taken, therefore, to use out-placement only when all other instructional attempts have failed to yield satisfactory results.

Prominent Instruments

As no standardized tests can be tailored to every specific curriculum, the academic achievement tests focus on basic skills included in any acceptable curriculum: reading skills (i.e., sounding out words, decoding, comprehension of the meaning of written material, reading speed, and skill at reading aloud), math skills (i.e., computational skills, reasoning skill used to solve word problems, and problem-solving efficiency), and written language skills (i.e., sentence construction and manipulation, essay composition and spelling, and knowledge of grammar). Academic achievement testing focuses on oral language skills, as well; typically, these tests examine a youngster's skill at both understanding oral communication and expressing themselves in oral language.

The Kaufman Test of Educational Achievement (KTEA-3; Kaufman & Kaufman, 2014) and the Wechsler Individual Achievement Test (WIAT-4; Wechsler, 2020) are the two main test batteries used to measure academic achievement. The tests vary somewhat in relation to age range, with the WIAT-4 (Wechsler, 2020) covering adults as well as children and adolescents and the KTEA-3 (Kaufman & Kaufman, 2014) covering only children and adolescents. The two measures also vary regarding specific academic skills assessed. Although each test measures core reading,

Table 1 Prominent instruments for assessing academic achievement

Test name and publication date	Age range	Information provided by test
Kaufman Test of Educational Achievement – Third Edition (KTEA-3) 2014	4 years, 0 months – 25 years, 11 months	Reading Math Written language Reading-related Oral Cross-domain
Wechsler Individual Achievement Test – Fourth Edition (WIAT-4) 2020	4 years, 0 months – 50 years, 11 months	Reading Basic reading Decoding Reading fluency Dyslexia index Written expression Writing fluency Mathematics Math fluency Oral language Phonological processing Orthographic processing Total achievement
Woodcock-Johnson IV Tests of Academic Achievement (WJ IV ACH) 2014	2 years – 90+ years	Reading Broad reading Basic reading skills Reading comprehension Reading fluency Reading rate Mathematics Broad mathematics Math calculation skills Math problem solving Written language Broad written language Basic writing skills Written expression Academic skills Academic fluency Academic applications Academic knowledge Phoneme-grapheme knowledge Brief or broad achievement
Kaufman Survey of Early Academic and Language Skills (K-SEALS) 1993	3 years, 0 months – 6 years, 11 months	Language skills Pre-academic skills Articulation

writing, math, and oral language skills, different associated skills are sampled on the two instruments. To customize a psychological assessment, psychologists often choose and combine particular subtests on the two batteries to ensure that an individual youngster is understood as completely as possible.

The Woodcock-Johnson IV Tests of Academic Achievement (WJ IV ACH; Mather & Wendling, 2014) are also a valuable instrument for examining scholastic accomplishments. Like the WIAT-4 (Wechsler, 2020) and the KTEA-3 (Kaufman & Kaufman, 2014), the WJ IV ACH (Mather & Wendling, 2014) also examines reading, math, and written language. Additionally, somewhat uniquely among tests of academic achievement, the WJ IV ACH (Mather & Wendling, 2014) can assess particular academic content areas (i.e., science, social studies, and humanities). While such assessment can be informative, interpretive caution is necessary. Since students in different educational settings are exposed to very different curricula and teaching methods, it is impossible to be certain whether scores in the content areas primarily reflect characteristics of youngsters or of their educational systems.

The assessment of very young children poses a singular challenge for academic achievement testing. Given their young age, they have yet to be exposed to much formal academic material and instruction. Thus, it would be unfair and irrelevant to test academic achievement in the same way that an older child or adolescent would be tested. However, in many cases, it is nevertheless important to obtain information about the strength of a youngster's foundation of pre-academic knowledge. The Kaufman Survey of Early Academic and Language Skills (K-SEALS; Kaufman & Kaufman, 1993) can be used to gather such information. Using a child-friendly, tabletop easel with bright pictures, the K-SEALS (Kaufman & Kaufman, 1993) measures receptive and expressive vocabulary, beginning mastery of quantitative concepts and number manipulation, and clarity of speech. K-SEALS (Kaufman & Kaufman, 1993) results are often a major asset in planning early intervention programs for preschool and primary school children (Table 1).

References

Kaufman, A. S., & Kaufman, N. L. (1993). *K-SEALS: Kaufman Survey of Early Academic and Language Skills*. American Guidance Service.

Kaufman, A. S., & Kaufman, N. L. (2014). *KTEA-3: Kaufman Test of Educational Achievement* (3rd ed.). Psychological Corporation.

Mather, N., & Wendling, B. J. (2014). *Woodcock-Johnson IV Tests of Academic Achievement* (4th ed.). Riverside.

Rakap, S., & Parlak-Rakap, A. (2011). Effectiveness of embedded instruction in early childhood special education: A literature review. *European Early Childhood Education Research Journal, 19*(1), 79–96. https://doi.org/10.1080/1350293X.2011.548946

Restori, A. F., Katz, G. S., & Lee, H. B. (2009). A critique of the IQ/Achievement Discrepancy Model for identifying specific learning disabilities. *Europe's Journal of Psychology, 5*(4). https://doi.org/10.5964/ejop.v5i4.244

Rotatori, A. F., Obiakor, F. E., & Bakken, J. P. (Eds.). (2011). *History of special education* (Vol. 21). Emerald Group Publishing Limited.

Wechsler, D. (2020). *WIAT-4: Wechsler Individual Achievement Test*. Psychological Corporation.

Behavioral Functioning

Basic Definitions

Behavioral functioning refers to the observable actions displayed by an individual. Behavioral problems – such as opposition to reasonable limits, school avoidance, excessive sibling conflict, and refusal to engage in age-appropriate peer interactions – often constitute an outcome of complex interactions among biological, developmental, and environmental factors. In many cases, these behavioral problems represent only the visible tip of more deeply-rooted social-emotional problems, which careful assessment can help examine and explain. (Please find additional information in the Social-Emotional Functioning chapter.)

Why Measure Behavioral Functioning?

Referral of a youngster for psychological testing often signifies that aspects of their behavior are viewed as inadequate or inappropriate. To know the best way to intervene, it is critical to determine the accuracy of this judgment. For accurate characterization of the youngster, it is extremely important to distinguish between subjective judgments of behavioral difficulty and objective data that verify the extent to which the youngster resembles or differs from most of their same-aged peers. Tests of behavioral functioning allow for such a distinction by providing information about the normative basis for concern about a youngster's behavior.

Determining the extent of behavioral difficulty then allows for appropriate forms of assistance to be offered. For example, behavioral functioning assessment results may indicate that there is a discrete behavioral disturbance that behavior modification would best address. In other instances, the results may

© Springer Nature Switzerland AG 2021   93
N. E. Moss, L. Moss-Racusin, *Practical Guide to Child and Adolescent Psychological Testing*, Best Practices in Child and Adolescent Behavioral Health Care, https://doi.org/10.1007/978-3-030-73515-9_14

indicate that an undesirable behavior is masking an underlying social-emotional concern best served by therapeutic assistance. In still other instances, the results may identify an environmental stressor that must be better managed to allow for a youngster's improved behavioral functioning. Results may also allow for the realization that adults judging a youngster's behavior are actually the most in need of assistance.

Common Patterns of Difficulty

There are many ways to organize and conceptualize the range of behavior problems seen in children and adolescents. For this book, behavior problems are considered to fall into one of three broad groups: internalizing, externalizing, and grossly inappropriate behaviors. Behavior problems in each of these groups can have a range of root causes.

Internalizing Behavior Problems

Nature of Difficulty   Problems in this domain are often associated with disorders such as anxiety and depression. Youngsters with internalizing behavior problems engage in inappropriate actions that threaten their own welfare. They direct their actions inward in ways that may damage their emotional wellbeing (e.g., overbooking themselves so as to avoid addressing a painful experience that needs to be processed), bodily integrity (e.g., self-injuring), and interpersonal connectedness (e.g., withdrawing from supportive relationships). They do not lash out at others, damage their physical environments, or engage in dangerous thrill-seeking activities. Their negative experiences are contained within them, as opposed to acted out.

Youth with internalizing behavior problems vary greatly in their experience of the behaviors and in their desire for assistance. Some youngsters are miserable and make repeated, powerful, overt and/or covert requests for help from those closest to them. Other youngsters are relatively unbothered by their problematic behaviors, and if left to themselves, would continue to engage in them. These youngsters become more overtly distressed only when their behaviors are interrupted, even when that interruption comes from caring adults and/or peers. The impact of internalizing behavior problems on those around a youth also varies. Adults may not be aware of the behaviors. If they are, they often become rightfully distraught in the face of manifestations of their youngster's problems, such as frequent weeping, scars, or repeated weekends without get-togethers with peers.

Externalizing Behavior Problems

Nature of Difficulty In this domain, behavior problems take the form of acting out. Youngsters with externalizing behavior problems can disrupt activities (e.g., yell loudly while a teacher is attempting to teach a lesson), damage property (e.g., break valued family keepsakes), endanger themselves (e.g., drive recklessly and excessively above the speed limit), and cause physical harm to other people (e.g., hit peers). As a result, they tend to face interpersonal isolation, frequent punishment, and sometimes even more dire consequences. Their self-esteem may also suffer significantly.

Psychological assessment findings can be very useful in characterizing externalizing behavior problems. Specifically, careful analysis of the results can determine whether an acting out behavior reflects a primary wish to oppose or hurt other people, or rather a primary need to express and discharge distress, however inappropriately. Being able to make this distinction allows for essential fine-tuning of interventions.

Grossly Inappropriate Behaviors

Nature of Difficulty Some children and adolescents display highly unusual behaviors that violate most people's expectations of reasonable responses to interpersonal interactions, situational demands, and environmental constraints. Examples of such grossly inappropriate behaviors include continuous repetition of non-communicative language and persistent, mechanical rocking back and forth. These extreme behaviors are manifested most typically by individuals with a significant Intellectual Disability, a major developmental disorder such as an Autism Spectrum Disorder, or an acute psychotic disorder.

How Do We Help?

Adult Understanding Effective behavior management rests on the assumption that all behavior has meaning; any behavior exhibited by a youngster conveys some important information. Worry about family wellbeing, unrelenting anxiety, fear and anger due to experiencing racism, inability to decipher a social cue, frustration due to a Learning Disorder, or lack of comprehension of a directive due to impaired intelligence are among the many underlying difficulties that could fuel inappropriate behavior. In fortunate cases, simple inquiry helps a youngster to share the source of their unacceptable behavior. Once this information is shared, appropriate steps can be taken to address the root problem, thereby eliminating the need to act inappropriately. Much more often, though, youngsters are unable to be so forthcoming. Typically, this inability is due not to an intentional withholding of necessary information, but rather to a genuine inability to identify the true cause of their undesirable behavior. In these more typical cases, it is the responsibility of the adults involved to examine the situation and continue exploring until the youngster's communication is comprehended. Armed with the knowledge of what a youngster is trying to convey, parents and caregivers can then determine whether some change can be carried out that, in effect, responds to the youngster's communication and removes the need to behave inappropriately.

As a professional, working toward behavior change for a youngster always begins with careful consultation with relevant adults. The most fundamental consultation is with parents and caregivers. Such consultation centers on learning about the youth's behavior and how the adults respond to it, as well as developing greater understanding of it. In some cases, ongoing consultation can help parents and caregivers to shift their own maladaptive responses to the youth in order to achieve a better outcome. For example, a preadolescent boy who hates to travel may be in a family that has the desire and means to travel extensively. Whenever the family plans or goes on a trip, he cries extensively, hurls insults at his parents, and does everything possible to sabotage the trip. The parents, with the best of intentions, keep trying to pick destinations they believe he will like and persist in pointing out to him all of the inviting features of their travel plans. However, this effort turns out to only make the boy feel profoundly misunderstood and alone, which fuels him to act out more. Building on this finding, parent consultation can then help the parents to better understand their son's reaction and to respond differently. They do not sacrifice their travel, but they explicitly acknowledge his feelings. They also learn to arrange trips with some unscheduled time built into each day for him to pursue solitary activities he likes, and they make sure to bring along his gaming materials. In the end, travel remains undesirable to the boy, but family vacations became much more peaceful for everyone.

When behavior problems manifest in school, teachers and related personnel should participate in ongoing consultation. Out of this consultation, structural and procedural changes can be suggested to make classroom settings and routines less conducive to inappropriate behaviors. To illustrate, an elementary school student may become noisy and oppositional whenever assignments are handed out. Assessment indicates that she is deeply afraid of making mistakes in her written work, so much so that she prefers to be in trouble rather than to submit an imperfect product. Consultation with her teacher then leads to the teacher giving her a required quota of mistakes to make each day. Once she fills her quota, she can receive a simple reward of her choosing. At first, the student is startled and disbelieving, but soon, making mistakes becomes a routine part of any effort, rather than a terrible disaster to be avoided at all costs. Her classroom behavior becomes calm and purposeful. After a time, the quota plan is faded out, no longer needed.

In attempting to help with child and adolescent behavior problems, another critical step is establishing adult understanding that behavior change requires organized effort. Adults' beliefs that youngsters should simply do as they are told, (possibly idealized) memories of their own obedience while growing up, preoccupation with other compelling life concerns, incomplete understanding of the behavioral implications of a youngster's diagnosis, lack of knowledge about how exactly to approach behavior management, as well as cultural emphasis on unquestioning respect for elders can all contribute to adults resorting to single-minded insistence that a youngster improve. Such insistence alone, however, typically only results in markedly frustrating power struggles and further behavioral deterioration by youngsters. It is critical to help adults understand that instead, creative and well-orchestrated approaches are the best opportunity for managing youngsters' behaviors and enjoying a more peaceful, harmonious life with them. Although adults may feel taxed by, and even resent, the need to work hard for behavior change, they can be assured that such work has the best chance of leading to attainment of their behavioral goals for their youngsters.

Environmental Interventions In many cases, elements in a youngster's environment inadvertently perpetuate behavior problems. Therefore, when psychological test findings identify specific behavior problems, it is always worthwhile to closely examine a youngster's environment for influences that may be giving rise to the problems. Direct observation of the youngster in their environment, in-depth conversation with the youngster, and detailed descriptions from trusted adults can assist with such examination. Then, when warranted, changing environmental conditions can often have a profound effect on behavior problems. To illustrate, a preschooler may have a great deal of trouble using the toilet in her home. When pushed to do so, her behavior becomes very disruptive to the entire family. Her parents request psychological assessment in order to get help bringing her behavior under control. Thorough evaluation and discussion reveal that the girl is terrified of the toilet water's unnatural shade of blue, the result of toilet bowl cleaner used by the family. When the family switches to a different toilet bowl cleaner, the girl's behavior problem evaporates.

Behavior Management Plans Understanding the communication behind inappropriate behaviors and making reasonable interpersonal and environmental accommodations are powerful tools in many cases. However, in others, unacceptable behaviors doggedly persist. Here, a behavior management plan should be constructed and implemented. The plan should be designed through collaboration between a youngster, relevant adults in their life, and professionals with expertise in responding to behavior problems. The youngster's participation is essential in order to ensure their understanding of the endeavor and to guarantee that sufficient motivation is built into the plan. Youngsters typically contribute honest, worthwhile suggestions. In the instances when their contributions are counterproductive or unrealistic, adults can retain veto power. Relevant adults need to participate to make sure that the plan is based on accurate knowledge of the youngster and the youngster's behavioral difficulties. Experts are needed so that the plan derives from sound principles of human behavior. A comprehensive behavior management plan should consist of the following components.

Identification of Target Behaviors A behavior management plan should be built on a recognition that true, meaningful behavior change is difficult to achieve. Real change requires painstaking effort. This effort has the greatest chance of success if it is directed at one, or at the most two, behaviors at a time. Trying to change multiple problematic behaviors at the same time tends to be overwhelming and lead to failure and discouragement for all involved. Adults often worry, though, that multiple, equally inappropriate behaviors are being left uncorrected while the behavior plan proceeds with its designated focus. Conversation with a youngster is useful here. In discussion, adults should be clear that other inappropriate behaviors also require attention, and that they will be addressed in due time, once everyone involved has some initial success on which to build.

Adults should choose target behaviors carefully. Usually, it is best to target the behaviors that are causing the most disruption in daily living. Reducing or eradicating the most disruptive behaviors provides the most powerful reward for effort expended, and thereby, also engenders the most motivation for broader behavior management efforts going forward. However, in cases where there is already considerable discouragement, it may be best to choose a less highly charged behavior, as it might be easier to change. Success, even in a limited sphere, can propel people forward to more confidently tackle larger behavior problems.

Behavioral Education Many adults assume that children and adolescents know very well which of their behaviors are inappropriate and what behaviors would be acceptable replacements. Contrary to this assumption, though, many youngsters do not actually have an accurate understanding of their misbehavior. They have even less understanding of what would constitute more appropriate behavior. To achieve success, a high quality behavior management plan rests on thorough instruction. It is impossible to be too specific or concrete in teaching children and adolescents how to distinguish between desirable and unacceptable behaviors. When teaching, in order to promote good interpersonal functioning, it is important to emphasize the impact of youngsters' behaviors on others. This emphasis helps youngsters learn how to behave in ways most likely to elicit a positive response from others.

Explicit Expectations Once target behaviors have been selected and youngsters have an adequate understanding of what constitutes desirable behavior, the next step is to set the clearest possible expectations for comportment. Content, setting, timing, duration, and requirements for repetition of the desired behavior should all be stipulated explicitly. Most importantly, standards for success should be spelled out with no room for misunderstanding. To maximize cooperation from the youngster, it is best for them to participate in the discussion that sets the expectations.

Specified Behavioral Supports Even with the best possible plan and cooperation from all involved, most youngsters need reminders and warnings in order to maximize their compliance with the plan. For a successful outcome, all involved should agree on whether or not prompts will be used in the plan, and if so, the form, number, and timing of them. Without specificity about behavioral supports, it is too easy for youngsters and adults to fall into pleading, bargaining, and endless repetitions of instructions. Adults and youngsters are usually successful in coming to agreement about behavioral supports in the plan.

Mutually Agreed Upon Rewards for Compliance Adults must be prepared to monitor their youngster's level of compliance with the behavior management plan. Ideally, youngsters would feel automatically inspired to comply with it. Absent inherent motivation, it would be wonderful if social approval from adults were a sufficient incentive for compliance. More realistic for many youngsters, though, is that tangible rewards are the most robust way to promote appropriate behavior (Payne & Dozier, 2013). The rewards should be mutually agreed upon by adults and youngsters, ensuring that they are indeed sufficiently desirable to motivate appropriate behavior. Children and adolescents will typically be honest about what rewards will be enticing enough to elicit their compliance. Often, the best choices involve games or items that have many parts. The parts can be given according to the behavior plan schedule, building toward the ultimate reward of having the full object of choice. Importantly, adults retain veto power about reward choice. Financial limitations and concerns about age appropriateness are relevant considerations in selecting rewards.

Mutually Agreed Upon Negative Consequences for Lack of Compliance While rewards are highly effective at increasing appropriate behavior (Payne & Dozier, 2013), there are cases in which youngsters must experience some form of penalty to reorient them toward appropriate behavior. Just as rewards should be mutually agreed upon, so too should negative consequences be. Again, most often, children and adolescents are frank about what consequences are so eagerly avoided that they will motivate appropriate behavior.

Several considerations are important in choosing negative consequences. First, they should be readily enforceable (e.g., reduced video game time). A consequence that depends too heavily on further cooperation from a youngster who is already behaving oppositionally (e.g., cleaning a room) simply plunges the adult and the youngster back into behavioral struggles. Second, consequences do not need to be severe or long to be effective. In fact, their severity and duration are far less important than the consistency with which they are administered. Children and adolescents learn best from reasonable, brisk, reliable negative consequences (Knox, 2010; Ma et al., 2012). Such consequences also avoid the pitfalls of youngsters resenting penalties they perceive as unfairly harsh and potentially trying to retaliate. Finally, negative consequences should be unpleasant for the youngster but not for the adult involved. Adults lose their own motivation to enforce consequences that interfere too extensively with their activities, and failing to consistently enforce consequences only extends and intensifies behavior problems.

Opportunities to Make Amends Individuals often seek to redeem themselves for wrongdoings, and doing so can be extremely reparative for all parties, as well as facilitative of more optimal functioning. Building opportunities into the behavior management plan for a youngster to make amends for inappropriate behavior provides similar benefits. The opportunities also elevate the plan above the level of simple rewards versus consequences, and teach youngsters how to enhance their interpersonal interactions. Offering a spontaneous and genuine apology, doing extra chores, and participating in a parent or caregiver's choice of leisure activity are all examples of ways to make amends for inappropriate behavior. It is then important for the recipient of the amends to acknowledge them.

Assessing When the Behavior Plan Is No Longer Necessary   A successful behavior management plan should become obsolete. The hope is that interpersonal, developmental, and self-esteem benefits of behaving more appropriately become powerful enough to sustain the desirable behavior. When appropriate behavior becomes more automatic, and the standards for success specified in the plan have been satisfied, it is reasonable to gradually discontinue use of the behavior management plan. A good signal that a plan can be relinquished is when a youngster who is consistently behaving well voices genuine confusion as to why their behavior plan is being continued. It should always be understood, though, that a plan can be reinstated, or a new one designed, whenever necessary.

Mental Health Interventions, Including Use of Medication   Sometimes, behavior problems persist despite adult support, environmental interventions, and use of a well-constructed behavior management plan. In these situations, further mental health treatment is indicated and may include use of psychiatric medication. More information about mental health interventions (including medication) that pertain to both behavioral and social-emotional functioning can be found in the Social-Emotional Functioning chapter.

Prominent Instruments

Behavioral measures are often in the form of checklists. Either the youngster themselves or an adult with extensive familiarity with the youngster responds to a set of statements about the youngster's behavior. Typically, the respondent indicates how often the designated behavior occurs, with ratings ranging from "Never" to "Almost Always." Specific behaviors are grouped to represent broad domains of behavior, as well as more well-defined subdomains. While behavioral test instruments vary somewhat, they typically focus on internalizing behaviors; externalizing behaviors; behaviors that reflect control over marshaling attention and sustaining concentration; frank behavioral problems; and more optimal, adaptive behaviors.

The Behavior Assessment System for Children (BASC-3; Reynolds et al., 2015) is a valued, comprehensive measure of behavioral functioning. It covers a wide age range and includes different forms to be completed by parents or caregivers, teachers, and also the youth being assessed. It is often useful to include multiple BASC-3 (Reynolds et al., 2015) forms in a comprehensive psychological assessment.

Table 1 Prominent instruments for assessing behavioral functioning

Test name and publication date	Age range	Information provided by test
Behavior Assessment System for Children – Third Edition (BASC-3) 2015	2 years, 0 months – 21 years, 11 months for teacher and parent rating scales	Adaptive and problem behaviors in the school setting, the home setting, and the community
	6 years, 0 months – college age for self-report of personality	Insight into thoughts and feelings

Comparison of reports on an individual's behavior from multiple perspectives can promote a richer, more nuanced understanding of a youngster's behavior in various circumstances. The BASC-3 (Reynolds et al., 2015) also includes a format for gathering comprehensive background information about a youngster (i.e., Structured Developmental History), as well as a carefully organized framework for formal observation of behavior (i.e., Student Observation System).

The BASC-3 (Reynolds et al., 2015) checklist format distinguishes first between clinical and adaptive behavior problems. On the Clinical Scale, the test further contrasts internalizing, distress-based behaviors with externalizing, acting out behaviors. The Clinical Scale also examines behavior problems related to inattention and academic functioning. On the Adaptive Scale, the test investigates an individual's facility with transitions, competence in navigating interpersonal interactions, ability to take the lead across situations, success at carrying out tasks required in everyday life, diligence as a student, and both engagement and accuracy in communicating with others. Summary scores are derived in each of these areas, along with an index of the extent to which negative emotions interfere in more optimal behavior. Given their different focus, the Structured Developmental History and Student Observation System each have their own unique format (Table 1).

References

Knox, M. (2010). On hitting children: A review of corporal punishment in the United States. *Journal of Pediatric Health Care, 24*(2), 103–107. https://doi.org/10.1016/j.pedhc.2009.03.001

Ma, J., Han, Y., Grogan-Kaylor, A., Delva, J., & Castillo, M. (2012). Corporal punishment and youth externalizing behavior in Santiago, Chile. *Child Abuse and Neglect, 36*(6), 481–490. https://doi.org/10.1016/j.chiabu.2012.03.006

Payne, S. W., & Dozier, C. L. (2013). Positive reinforcement as treatment for problem behavior maintained by negative reinforcement. *Journal of Applied Behavior Analysis, 46*(3), 699–703. https://doi.org/10.1002/jaba.54

Reynolds, C. R., Kamphaus, R. W., & Vannest, K. J. (2015). *BASC-3: Behavior Assessment System for Children.* Psychological Corporation.

Adaptive Behavior

Basic Definitions

Adaptive behavior refers to the range of skills each individual has in order to meet the demands of everyday life. The adaptive behavior domain of psychological testing evaluates the acquisition and demonstration of these skills in a variety of day-to-day situations and settings. Adaptive behaviors typically include a youngster's self-care, use of leisure time, fine and gross motor skills, sensitivity and responsibility, oral and written communication, social interactions, contributions to a household, community-oriented daily living skills (e.g., use of money, following traffic signals), and the extent of intrusiveness of undesirable, maladaptive behaviors that impede more optimal functioning.

Why Measure Adaptive Behavior?

Most broadly, tests of adaptive behavior allow for understanding of the quality and success of a youth's everyday living. They offer a clear snapshot of a youth's competence level in navigating daily life demands. Such a snapshot is an invaluable supplement to the results in other assessment domains. For example, it can demonstrate the extent to which a youth is able to use their intellectual abilities and academic skills to enhance their daily life.

More particularly, findings about adaptive behavior are necessary to support the identification of some diagnoses. Primary among these diagnoses is Intellectual Disability; impaired adaptive behavior is a core element required for its assignment. Moreover, providing clear evidence of deficient adaptive behavior to a state government is critical for obtaining essential health, educational, vocational, and housing services.

© Springer Nature Switzerland AG 2021

N. E. Moss, L. Moss-Racusin, *Practical Guide to Child and Adolescent Psychological Testing*, Best Practices in Child and Adolescent Behavioral Health Care, https://doi.org/10.1007/978-3-030-73515-9_15

Assessing adaptive behavior is also important, because it is a singularly important determinant of long-term quality of life. Regardless of the severity of a youngster's clinical diagnosis, any enhancement of their adaptive behavior eases their daily struggles. To illustrate, an older adolescent male with a severe Intellectual Disability may only be able to engage in a limited amount of activity and social interaction. However, he does learn to do laundry. Once he acquires this skill, he does his family's weekly laundry and enjoys the activity very much. This development in his adaptive behavior fills his days and enhances his mood.

A final reason to assess adaptive behavior is that proficiency in it is a major contributor to a youngster's self-esteem. The young child who is proud to tie their shoes without help, and the adolescent who takes satisfaction from cooking dinner for their family are examples of how youngsters' self-esteem can be strengthened through good adaptive skills.

Common Patterns of Difficulty

Inadequate Fulfillment of Daily Life Demands

Nature of Difficulty Psychological testing may reveal that a youngster has globally deficient adaptive behavior, meaning that they struggle with daily living skills, motor skills, management of logistics, socialization, and communication. Such a youngster would experience significantly reduced self-sufficiency. In other cases, test results can reveal specific domains of impaired adaptive skills (e.g., poor personal hygiene, lack of knowledge about how to navigate a stairway, difficulty requesting information, poor skill at interpreting whether peer groups are conveying a welcoming or rejecting message). These youngsters would also experience reduced self-sufficiency, but in circumscribed areas.

It is important to note that low scores on measures of adaptive behavior are not always reflective of weakness on the part of a youngster. Sometimes, they may reflect environmental constraints. If an individual is to have an adaptive skill, their environment must provide opportunities for it to be learned and carried out, and such opportunities are truly absent from some individuals' environments. In such situations, interpretation of test findings should note the absence of specified skills, but also emphasize that the absence is not representative of a youngster's adaptive weakness. For example, children and adolescents in a town so small that traffic can be managed without any lights would not be familiar with them or demonstrate obedience to them. However, lack of this adaptive skill reflects an environmental idiosyncrasy, not a personal limitation.

There are also situations in which the broad environment has opportunities to learn and do the full range of designated adaptive skills, but parents and caregivers do not allow youngsters to attempt them. In these situations, an adult's decision to prevent attempts at certain skills is generally understood as concern and realization that a youngster would be unable to do the skills safely and competently. Therefore, this type of skill absence can be interpreted as an adaptive weakness on the part of the youngster. To illustrate, a parent may purposely place the family microwave out of a youth's reach in order to avoid possible fire danger or another mishap. Placement of the microwave reflects that the youth lacks the skill to operate it, rather than an overall environmental limitation.

It is also important to note that sometimes, psychological test results indicate surprisingly good adaptive behavior. Some individuals, regardless of carrying severe mental health diagnoses, manage to gain impressive adaptive skills. For example, an adolescent with an Intellectual Disability may make their own dinner before a parent's return home. For these youngsters, it is critical to verify the accuracy of their mental health diagnoses. It is possible that their above-expected adaptive behavior signals erroneous diagnoses. If the diagnoses are confirmed, though, it is a reminder that a serious mental health diagnosis does not necessarily preclude the possibility of success and satisfaction. To help these youngsters move forward, all adults involved in their lives should exert maximum effort to support their continued growth and the refinement of their adaptive behavior.

How Do We Help? Unlike other capabilities (e.g., intellectual) that have inborn limitations in their responsiveness to intervention, adaptive behavior can almost always be improved. Even those individuals with very significant, comprehensive impairment can usually be taught to improve their adaptive skills. Improved adaptive behavior is a great source of enhanced self-esteem and quality of life.

In many domains, weaknesses identified through psychological testing require professional intervention in order to improve. In the adaptive behavior domain, though, parents and caregivers who are part of a youngster's daily life are typically the most effective at assisting with improvement. While they may benefit from professional guidance about how to best focus their efforts, they tend to have the greatest motivation, proximity, and knowledge of the youngster and of what can help bring about changes in the youngster's adaptive behavior.

Effective intervention in a youngster's adaptive behavior begins with an inventory of the daily functions designated as age-appropriate for them but currently being carried out by their parents or caregivers on their behalf. Adults are then asked to identify which of these functions, if taken over by their youngster, would provide them with the greatest relief. Focusing on a function with the greatest potential to ease an adult's daily routine maximizes their motivation to engage in teaching their youngster a new adaptive skill.

The specified skill is then identified to the youngster, who should be reassured that no criticism is intended, and that rather, teaching them a new skill is intended to increase their mastery and pride. The skill is explained in detail and demonstrated as many times as necessary. Questions and comments are encouraged from the youngster. Once the youngster indicates that they understand the skill, it is time for them to attempt it under adult supervision. In a non-judgmental way, the adult can offer constructive criticism and guidance to refine the youngster's performance. Once both adult and youngster are confident that the skill has been acquired and can be optimally enacted, the adult's presence can be withdrawn gradually. Adult assistance can always be reintroduced if the youngster experiences difficulty in carrying out a skill.

It is important to clearly inform adults that many repetitions and trials will likely be required for optimal skill acquisition by their youngster. A common objection from adults about adaptive behavior training concerns the amount of teaching effort that is required. They will often protest that they just want free time to relax after extensive work hours and/or other responsibilities. While disliking the sacrifice of free time to take on instruction in adaptive behavior is understandable, it overlooks the ongoing discomfort and intrusiveness of having to make up for inadequacies in youngsters' adaptive behavior. It can be useful to point out that time-limited teaching effort, while sometimes strenuous, typically yields long-lasting and significant rewards (i.e., a better chance of leisure). Furthermore, success in gaining one new adaptive skill tends to facilitate additional success. Both adults and youngsters are usually highly pleased by the success, which in turn propels them to tackle more adaptive skills with heightened motivation, confidence, and competence.

Prominent Instruments

Tests of adaptive behavior are rarely completed by the individual being assessed. Rather, they are usually completed by respondents who have close, full-time familiarity with the individual. These respondents (e.g., parents, caregivers, teachers) are in a good position to be able describe the daily adaptive skills displayed by the individual.

The Vineland Adaptive Behavior Scales (Vineland-3; Sparrow et al., 2016) are the chief, highest quality measure of adaptive behavior. Their first iteration was called the Vineland Social Maturity Scale (Doll, 1947) and was the first to recognize management of daily life challenges as an appropriate focus of assessment. Although standardized on a relatively small, unique population, the test proved very useful and was widely used. Several decades later, the test was revised dramatically and was renamed the Vineland Adaptive Behavior Scales (Sparrow & Doll, 1984). Much of the format changed, item analysis and design modernized the content of the test, and statistical underpinnings were updated to conform to more currently accepted methodological standards. The Vineland Adaptive Behavior Scales (Sparrow & Doll, 1984) were revised twice after that. In each revision, structural enhancements were made, and items were updated.

Item updates are critical for measures of adaptive behavior to remain helpful. Items must reflect progress and change in technology, cultural practices, and community standards if the results are to be accepted as accurate measures of adaptive behavior. Given the fast pace of societal change, it is a major challenge to ensure that measures of adaptive behavior remain sufficiently current.

Prominent alternatives to the Vineland-3 (Sparrow et al., 2016) are the Child Behavior Checklists for youth ages one-and-a-half to five (CBCL/1½-5; Achenbach

& Rescorla, 2000) and six to eighteen (CBCL/6-18; Achenbach, 2001). The CBCL/1½–5 (Achenbach & Rescorla, 2000) and CBCL/6-18 (Achenbach, 2001) are part of a more comprehensive behavioral assessment system: the Achenbach System of Empirically Based Assessment (ASEBA). The ASEBA uses checklists for parents and caregivers, teachers, and youths themselves to gather information on multiple areas of behavioral functioning across the life span. The CBCL/1½–5 (Achenbach & Rescorla, 2000) and CBCL/6-18 (Achenbach, 2001) specifically assess adaptive behavior through parent and caregiver reports. As test instruments, they are subject to the same constraints described in relation to the Vineland-3 (Sparrow et al., 2016) (Table 1).

Table 1 Prominent instruments for assessing adaptive behavior

Test name and publication date	Age range	Information provided by test
Vineland Adaptive Behavior Scales – Third Edition (Vineland-3) 2016	Birth – 90 years	Communication: Receptive Expressive Written
		Daily living skills: Personal Domestic Community
		Socialization: Interpersonal relationships Play and leisure Coping skills
		Motor skills: Fine Gross
		Maladaptive behavior: Internalizing Externalizing
Child Behavior Checklist – Ages 1½–5 (CBCL/1½–5) 2000	1 year, 6 months – 5 years, 11 months	Syndrome scales: Emotionally reactive Anxious/depressed Somatic complaints Withdrawn Sleep problems Attention problems Aggressive behavior Stress problems
		DSM-oriented scales: Depressive problems Anxiety problems Autism Spectrum problems Attention-Deficit/Hyperactivity problems Oppositional defiant problems Language development survey

(continued)

Table 1 (continued)

Test name and publication date	Age range	Information provided by test
Child Behavior Checklist – Ages 6-18 (CBCL/6-18) 2001	6 years – 18 years	Syndrome scales: Anxious/depressed Depressed Somatic complaints Social problems Thought problems Attention problems Rule-breaking behavior Aggressive behavior
		DSM-oriented scales: Affective problems Anxiety problems Somatic problems Attention-Deficit/Hyperactivity problems Oppositional defiant problems Conduct problems
		Competence scales: Activities Social relations School Total competence
		Obsessive Compulsive Disorder scale Posttraumatic Stress Disorder scale

References

Achenbach, T. (2001). *Child Behavior Checklist, Ages 6–18*. ASEBA.

Achenbach, T., & Rescorla, L. (2000). *Child Behavior Checklist, Ages 1½–5*. ASEBA.

Doll, E. A. (1947). *Vineland Social Maturity Scale: Condensed Manual of Directions*. Educational Test Bureau, Educational Publishers.

Sparrow, S. S., & Doll, E. A. (1984). *Vineland Adaptive Behavior Scales*. AGS.

Sparrow, S. S., Cicchetti, D. V., Saulnier, C. A., & Doll, E. A. (2016). *Vineland-3: Vineland Adaptive Behavior Scales* (3rd ed.). Psychological Corporation.

Social-Emotional Functioning

Basic Definitions

Social-emotional functioning pertains to the manifestations of a youngster's internal emotional life. Capacity to participate socially, ability to adhere to social norms while engaged with others, and degree of comfort in interpersonal interactions are all important components of the social aspects of this domain. The emotional aspects include the nature, intensity, regulation, and correspondence to the external environment of a youngster's feelings. Social-emotional functioning can be further understood in relation to the following domains.

Issues of Concern to the Youngster

Children and adolescents commonly identify struggles at school, social disappointments, and family discord as areas of concern. At times, a youngster's report of concerns is entirely consistent with an adult's, in which case there is helpful consensus about problems to tackle. Many other times, though, a youngster's report is either an underestimate of their difficulties, possibly for defensive reasons, or an exaggeration of their difficulties, possibly representing unduly harsh self-criticism. At all times, understanding a youngster's viewpoint regarding their concerns provides useful insight into the youngster and a good index of their capacity and likelihood to productively participate in interventions.

© Springer Nature Switzerland AG 2021
N. E. Moss, L. Moss-Racusin, *Practical Guide to Child and Adolescent
Psychological Testing*, Best Practices in Child and Adolescent Behavioral
Health Care, https://doi.org/10.1007/978-3-030-73515-9_16

Self-Concept/Self-Esteem and Interpersonal Relationships

A youngster's relationships with themselves and with other people are important components of social-emotional functioning. Some youngsters note these domains as areas of concern. Some youngsters do not, but parents, caregivers, teachers, and providers note them to be. A youngster's sense of self, the degree to which they accurately assess their strengths and problem areas, and the extent to which they engage in self-approval and/or punitive self-criticism are all relevant to social-emotional wellbeing. As for interpersonal relationships, it is essential to note if a youngster experiences them as a resource for solving problems and feeling better, or as toxic and destructive. It is equally essential to assess the alignment between a youngster's appraisal of their relationships and how those relationships actually are. The closer the alignment, the more optimism is warranted about a youngster's eventual outcomes.

Feelings

Youngsters always have emotions relevant to their identified concerns, but they can differ in their awareness and expression of these emotions. Sometimes, some of their feelings may be conveyed directly (e.g., a youth describes sadness about a deceased relative or voices anger at a sibling). Other times, some of their feelings have to be inferred from less direct behaviors. These feelings can be understood as having an impact on a youngster's functioning but remaining largely outside of their awareness. For example, an adolescent might speak to a peer, in whom they are romantically interested, using long, pressured, and disorganized phrases. Such speech could suggest that the adolescent feels nervous.

Coping Strategies

Youngsters vary in how equipped they are to deal with their concerns and related feelings. Coping strategies employed by a child or adolescent can be divided into two main types. The first type is useful, instrumental action with encouraging potential for resolving a problematic issue or relieving an uncomfortable emotion (e.g., engaging in vigorous physical exercise to combat feelings of depression). The second type is less purposeful action with limited potential for success (e.g., provoking a furious argument with a caregiver to divert attention away from shame regarding difficulty focusing attention). Generally, the former type of problem-solving attempts call for encouragement, and the latter call for instruction in order to help identify more appropriate efforts.

Integrity of Reality Testing

The concerns a youngster notes, their associated feelings, and their coping skills all relate to their reality testing. Reality testing refers to the accuracy of environmental perceptions and the relative soundness of logical thinking. The hope is always that a youngster is able to understand reality accurately and respond to it skillfully. Such reality testing ability justifies optimism about ultimate outcomes, as noted above in the section on intra- and interpersonal relationships. When a youngster's reality testing is weak or frankly impaired, hopes for significant improvement have to be much more modest.

Why Measure Social-Emotional Functioning?

Put most simply, the social-emotional functioning portion of a comprehensive test battery provides vital information about how a youngster feels. This information is critical to an accurate understanding of a youngster. Findings about a youngster's emotional and interpersonal condition inform caregivers and professionals about a youngster's view of themselves developmentally, affectively, cognitively, socially, academically, and medically. Often, the findings provide a solid foundation for diagnosing. Based on the findings, interventions can be delivered in a way that is most sensitive to a youngster's emotional state and needs. Such individualized interventions have the most potential for success in providing true assistance to a youngster in need of help.

Common Patterns of Difficulty

A comprehensive discussion of all possible social-emotional difficulties present in childhood and adolescence is beyond the scope of this book. For this book, it is most appropriate to highlight the difficulties that are often detected or confirmed by psychological testing of youngsters.

Anxiety

Nature of Difficulty One prominent problem notable on psychological testing is anxiety. Identification of anxiety signifies that, even absent genuine danger, a youngster is bothered by excessive and often unrealistic worry that is either generalized or focused on specific settings, activities, people, or bodily sensations (American Psychiatric Association, 2013). A child in a constant state of apprehension about separation from their caregivers, and an adolescent who is nervously preoc-cupied for months about having to give a class presentation are both examples of individuals who would likely merit a diagnosis of an anxiety disorder.

Depression

Nature of Difficulty Another problem often detected by psychological assessment is depression. Children and adolescents with depression tend to display some com-bination of low mood, helplessness, hopelessness, irritability, limited energy and motivation, altered sleep and appetite, and loss of capacity to take pleasure in activi-ties that were previously enjoyable. Some youngsters with depression may also engage in self-injury and/or have suicidal ideation (American Psychiatric Association, 2013). A child who retreats to their room, spending long, solitary hours lying listlessly on their bed, or an adolescent who responds to any conversational overtures by caregivers with hostile retorts are examples of youngsters struggling with depression.

Depression can be a distinct, unipolar disorder or a feature of Bipolar Disorder. Some manifestations of Bipolar Disorder involve alternation between depression and mania or hypomania. Hypomanic and manic states can include activity levels that are excessive but rarely truly productive; impulsivity; grandiosity; extremely poor self-regulation; irritability, anger flare-ups, and interpersonal conflict; inability to relax or sleep, or belief that doing so is personally unnecessary; and unrealistic and inappropriate thinking and speech. Hypomanic states are less severe versions of manic states. Bipolar Disorder is diagnosed rarely and extremely cautiously in young children, as course of development remains largely unclear. It can be diag-nosed more confidently among older children and adolescents (American Psychiatric Association, 2013).

Trauma

Nature of Difficulty Psychological testing can also indicate trauma. At times, responses to test instruments may allow for initial identification of a trauma experi-enced by a child or adolescent. For example, sexually suggestive responses can alert a psychologist to assess for possible sexual abuse, which may not have been recog-nized previously. More typically, though, a youngster's trauma experience is discov-ered through other means (e.g., direct observation by others, self-report by the youngster, or medical appointments). In these more common cases, social-emotional test instruments then serve to help gauge the impact of trauma on the youngster's developmental progression, physiological functioning, self-regulation, emotional wellbeing, reality testing, and interpersonal relationships. For example, analysis of social-emotional assessment results for an adolescent who lashes out dangerously at their child welfare caseworker may establish a direct link between their longstanding physical abuse and their poorly regulated behavior and struggle to trust even helpful adults.

Psychosis

Nature of Difficulty The utility of psychological testing is also noteworthy in relation to psychosis. Fundamentally, a psychotic disorder is one in which reality testing is significantly impaired. Unusual, inaccurate, illogical, and disorganized environmental perceptions, statements, and behaviors observed throughout assessment may suggest psychosis. A child who insists that their parent is lying on the floor of a psychologist's office, and the adolescent who cries out of worry they are transforming into the monster they have been "seeing" roaming their school hallways exemplify young people with psychosis.

How Do We Help?

There is a range of possible interventions for addressing social-emotional problems. They are not mutually exclusive, and often, it is most helpful to recommend a combination of them.

Psychoeducation can lay the foundation to productively remediate social-emotional difficulties. Clear, truthful, developmentally-attuned information about the challenges, and possibly the disorders, with which youngsters are contending can reassure them that they are facing known phenomenon. Adults offering names and explanations for their problems unequivocally conveys that the problems are not mysterious, dangerous unknowns without possibility for improvement. Empathic sharing of information can also demonstrate that many people experience a given problem or diagnosis. Realizing that they are not alone provides a measure of relief to most children and adolescents. Additionally, psychoeducation can protect youngsters' self-esteem by clarifying that mental health problems are the result of combined heredity and environmental experience (Tsuang et al., 2004; Uher & Zwicker, 2017), rather than of any personal flaw. Finally, psychoeducation can ready a youngster to understand and cooperate with interventions on their behalf.

Many caring adults worry that psychoeducation in relationship to social-emotional problems will be devastating to a young person's sense of self. They are concerned that the youngster will perceive themselves as hopelessly damaged if informed and educated about their difficulties. In actuality, though, most youngsters are rarely surprised by the psychoeducational information. Typically, they have been struggling with the experience and consequences of their difficulties for a long time, without the benefit of fully understanding what was happening to them. With good psychoeducation, they can finally understand, and hopefully also experience the other benefits described above. Having received accurate psycho-education, youngsters (and the adults in their lives) may feel sad and angry that they have to manage a particular problem or disorder, and these emotions are reasonable. With sufficient clinical empathy and support, though, youngsters and their caregivers can move toward greater acceptance and engagement in therapeutic interventions.

One such intervention is to teach children and adolescents various coping strategies that can bring significant relief of symptoms and distress. Deep breathing techniques, different methods for practicing mindfulness, meditation, yoga, physical exercise, designated leisure activities, empowering affirmations, and visualization of positive experiences are all examples of such strategies. Youngsters are taught to recognize the onset of distress episodes and to implement their strategies in these moments in order to help themselves return to a state of greater emotional equilibrium. Youngsters are also taught to implement ongoing regulatory strategies, such as structured daily routines, in order to minimize the occurrence of distress episodes in the first place. Relatedly, many children and adolescents with social-emotional problems benefit from participation in activities that provide peer interaction, community connection, skill acquisition, and fun. As long as leaders are able to accommodate these youngsters (e.g., by allowing a caregiver to sit in quietly, by permitting a distressed youngster to take a break and then return when ready), music lessons and performance, art instruction, gaming clubs, swimming lessons, gymnastics, martial arts, therapeutic horseback riding, scouting, and faith-based youth groups all exemplify activities that can enhance their lives.

There are also many types of formal mental health treatment for children and adolescents who struggle socially-emotionally. Several of them are listed and briefly described below. Formal treatment is recommended when social-emotional problems cause pervasive and significant psychological distress, raise the realistic possibility of harm to self or others, impair a youngster's daily functioning, and/or are unlikely to improve without professional guidance, all of which can be determined by assessment findings.

When recommending formal mental health treatment, evaluating psychologists should avoid suggesting treatments that have already been attempted, unless they are being suggested with a substantive difference. Some psychologists are highly specific in their recommendations, providing detailed instructions about how treatment should proceed. Such recommendations may be useful but also risk offending the therapists who receive them. This offense can ultimately hurt a youngster by inserting a barrier in their treatment. Other psychologists make broader recommendations for types and overall goals of treatment. These recommendations avoid the risk of offense but may require greater effort from the therapists. Thus, there are benefits and drawbacks to either approach.

Individual Psychodynamic Psychotherapy for the Youngster An assumption of this type of therapy is that the main therapeutic instrument is the alliance between youngster and therapist. Using the alliance, along with developmentally appropriate means (e.g., play for younger children, more discussion for older children and adolescents), therapist and youngster explore the psychological and emotional roots of presenting problems. Relevant thoughts and feelings are examined, and links are made between internal experiences and concrete behaviors. Over the course of treatment, as inner conflicts are explored and resolved, more appropriate behavioral patterns are also recommended and practiced.

Individual Cognitive Behavioral Therapy for the Youngster The primary assumption of this form of therapy is that emotional and behavioral struggles result from maladaptive thoughts. The mechanism of treatment is to clarify the links between problematic beliefs and undesirable feelings and actions, and then to adopt more healthful beliefs and behaviors, which can both, in turn, enhance emotional wellbeing. Ongoing treatment focuses on helping a youngster to practice and refine their newly acquired cognitive and behavioral skills.

Parent and Caregiver Counseling Children and adolescents almost always need their parents and caregivers to be involved in their psychological treatment, if it is to provide the maximum benefit. These adults typically have invaluable information about a youngster's daily life, so their contributions can ensure that a therapist is sufficiently informed and able to focus therapy on the most pressing needs.

As the therapist works with the youngster and helps the youngster develop skills, information can also be provided *to* the adults (in accordance with regulations and laws regarding confidentiality and privacy) in order to deepen their understanding of their youngster, guide their efforts to help their youngster, and enhance their family relationships. Parent and caregiver counseling helps them to respond supportively to, and reinforce, their youngster's efforts to change. It offers a place for them to do their own learning relevant to their youngster's wellbeing and to ask questions. Of note, there are also cases in which parent and caregiver counseling reveals psychological difficulties in the adults, who may require or benefit from their own separate treatment.

Family Therapy When psychological testing indicates that systemic problems within a family are major sources of a youth's difficulties, family therapy is typically recommended. Examples of family system problems include poor communication patterns, overly rigid or overly loose interpersonal boundaries, and high levels of conflict. Working with a specially trained therapist can help a family bring problems out into the open, learn skills to productively work through these problems, and create improved ways to interact that support each family member as fully as possible.

Group Therapy The assumption that underlies all therapeutic group endeavors is that immediate, shared, thoughtful experience can have a reparative impact. Beyond that, there are several types of groups with different emphases, and psychological assessment results can help pinpoint the type that can best address particular social-emotional problems.

Groups can be primarily supportive, aimed at lessening feelings of isolation and increasing validation and mutual understanding for youngsters navigating specific life challenges. A group for siblings of individuals with serious mental illness is an example of a support group.

Groups can also be primarily educational or skills-based, aimed at providing youngsters with instructive guidance in understanding and managing specific difficulties. Such groups typically incorporate the teaching and practicing of skills. Educational groups also have a supportive component, since they demonstrate to participants that others face similar struggles. A group for children with a common diagnosis (e.g., diabetes, an anxiety disorder) is an example of an educational group. A particular kind of educational group is a social skills group. A social skills group helps address the impacts of a range of social-emotional difficulties that can detract from a youngster's peer relationships and leisure activities. Social skills groups will be discussed further in the Developmental Status chapter.

Behavioral groups are another option for youngsters. These groups target specific behavioral problems. Using principles of behavioral analysis, the goal is to help group members adopt more acceptable behaviors. Intermittently explosive behavioral outbursts are an example of the kind of problem that can be addressed in a behavioral group. Group members' reflections on one another's struggles and progress can propel therapeutic progress.

Therapy groups differ on what, if any, contact they allow between members outside of meetings. These differences are due to safety and privacy considerations, type of group, style and theoretical orientation of the group leaders, and preferences of the group members and their caregivers. When contact is appropriate, therapy groups can be a source of new friendships, in addition to the benefits already listed.

Group therapy can be helpful as a stand-alone treatment modality or in combination with other forms of therapy. When combined with other therapies, the providers involved do best when they are in contact with each other (with legal permission) and collaborate and clarify which therapeutic tasks will be tackled in which therapy setting.

School-Based Counseling Services Some youngsters' social-emotional problems are rooted in or manifest most in the school setting. While therapeutic interventions outside of school can have a beneficial effect in such cases, school-based services (when available) are often able to address these problems more immediately and directly. "Lunch bunches," as school personnel often label their therapeutic groups; regularly scheduled individual counseling with a school mental health professional; and as needed crisis intervention in the school setting are all useful forms of school-based services. The school psychologists, school social workers, and guidance counselors who provide these services typically have a wealth of information about various situations a youngster faces at school and about the school environment. They also have the benefits of proximity to the youngster, availability in the moment, and direct access to school supports and resources that can be marshaled to address social-emotional problems. Another benefit of school-based services compared to non-school-based services is that a youngster's memory for school experiences and capacity for self-report, both of which can be limited, are less of a potential impediment to therapeutic progress.

Medication Psychiatric medication may be considered in regard to social-emotional difficulties. Typically, the idea of medication is introduced when social-emotional problems have a biological basis and/or when other efforts and interventions alone have not sufficiently reduced distress and improved functioning. Medication properly chosen and administered can be markedly helpful in such situations. Indeed, there is strong research support for the effectiveness of psychiatric medication in combination with therapy (e.g., Cuijpers et al., 2014).

Psychologists have ample training and experience in assessing and treating psychological difficulties using many techniques. As such, they can often develop a keen sense for when medication should be considered. In some instances, they may even have a solid sense of which medication or class of medication would be helpful. It is critical to emphasize, though, that psychologists are not medically trained, although some may choose to pursue training in pharmacology (American Psychological Association Services, Inc., 2014). The intricacies of possible interactions among particular medications and health conditions are outside the bounds of most psychological training. Therefore, most assessing psychologists recommend consultation with a medical professional when the option of using psychiatric medication arises.

Prominent Instruments

Several tests are widely used in this domain. These include the Machover Draw-a-Person Test (DAP; Machover, 1949), Kinetic Family Drawing (KFD; Burns & Kaufman, 1971), Rotter Incomplete Sentences Blank (RISB-2; Rotter et al., 1992), Thematic Apperception Test (TAT; Murray, 1971), Roberts Apperception Test for Children: 2 (Roberts-2; Roberts, 2005), Rorschach Test (Rorschach, 2014), and Structured Interview for Prodromal Syndromes (SIPS; McGlashan et al., 2001). Findings on each test make unique contributions to an overall social-emotional understanding of a youngster.

On the DAP (Machover, 1949), the youngster is asked to draw a whole person. They are free to choose all of the particulars in the drawing as long as a whole human being is presented. Once the first drawing is completed, the youngster is asked to draw a second whole person of another gender. It should be noted that, in the face of twenty-first century transformations in concepts and practices related to gender identity, a growing number of youngsters have begun to decline to label their human figures as either male or female. Psychologists must accommodate in their interpretations of test findings.

On the KFD (Burns & Kaufman, 1971), the youngster is asked to draw all the members of their family doing something. Again, all the particulars of the drawing are under the youngster's control. Since both the DAP (Machover, 1949) and the KFD (Burns & Kaufman, 1971) are purely visual, the youngster is often able to express thoughts, feelings, and concerns that would be too difficult to communicate in a more direct verbal exchange. The psychologist may ask some clarifying questions about the drawings, and later analyzes them in relation to the issues that prompted the assessment. Results on these measures often help to generate hypotheses about a youth's self-concept, social-emotional state, and view of others. These hypotheses are then confirmed or disconfirmed by other test findings. Many times, DAP (Machover, 1949) and KFD (Burns & Kaufman, 1971) findings also provide a clear, visual representation of complex issues that emerge in lengthier, more detailed forms on other social-emotional test instruments. This visual representation often streamlines and intensifies understanding of the youngster.

On the RISB-2 (Rotter et al., 1992), the youngster is presented with a relatively long list of sentence stems. They are asked to complete each sentence in any way they wish. The only rule is that the sentences must be true about them. Within the psychological test battery, the main contribution of the RISB-2 (Rotter et al., 1992) findings is identification of interests, wishes, thoughts, concerns, worries, and problems that are within the youngster's awareness. Such identification provides invaluable insight into the youngster's perspective and helps adults tailor intervention plans to actually address issues that matter most to the youngster.

The TAT (Murray, 1971) is a storytelling test. It is made up of a large group of pictures. The pictures depict people and objects, but the exact nature of their content is purposely unclear. To complete the test, a youngster is presented with a subset of the TAT (Murray, 1971) pictures and is asked to tell a story about each one. The psychologist either takes verbatim notes or records the individual telling their story. Again, the individual being assessed is in complete control of the story's content, except that they must include an explanation of each character's feelings and describe a clear ending. Analysis of the stories is primarily useful for learning about the youngster in relationship to others. Self-esteem and self-confidence in relationships, trust that others can be helpful, family discord, and distortion of interpersonal relationships are examples of issues about which the TAT (Murray, 1971) findings can be illuminating.

While still a very useful test with a rich clinical history, the TAT (Murray, 1971) does dates from around the mid-twentieth century. Newer apperception tests, such as the Roberts-2 (Roberts, 2005), have been constructed to elicit similar social-emotional data. On one hand, the newer test instruments have the advantage of conforming to more current standards regarding test design. On the other hand, they present pictures that depict more concrete and discernable plots than those on the TAT (Murray, 1971). As a result, youngsters may tend to provide stories that plainly describe the pictures rather than reveal their own underlying personality dynamics and emotions. Therefore, psychologists make thoughtful decisions about which apperception instruments to use with specific youngsters.

The Rorschach Test (Rorschach, 2014) examines the foundation of personality structure. The youngster is shown 10 cards, one at a time, each with a picture of an inkblot on it. The psychologist asks the youngster to relate what the inkblot might be and encourages the youngster to state more than one response. In a second phase of test administration, the youngster is asked to locate what they saw on the inkblot and then to describe what features of the inkblot contributed to their perception. As on the TAT (Murray, 1971), the psychologist makes note of all of the youngster's responses. Intricate scoring systems have been designed over the years to analyze Rorschach (Rorschach, 2014) responses. The Exner Scoring System (Exner, 2009) has the best empirical support and is the most widely used.

It is important to note that there is tremendous controversy about the reliability and validity of the Rorschach (Rorschach, 2014). Supporters of the test view it as providing unparalleled insight into the deepest levels of personality functioning. Critics dismiss the test as being unscientific, having unacceptably subjective scoring methods, and making potentially damaging statements about individuals without

Table 1 Prominent instruments for assessing social-emotional functioning

Test name and publication date.	Age range	Information provided by test
Machover Draw-a-Person Test (DAP) 1949	Unspecified	Perceptions of and feelings about self and interactions with social environment
Kinetic Family Drawing (KFD) 1971	Unspecified	Perceptions of and feelings about family structure, family connectedness, and sentient environment
Rotter Incomplete Sentences Blank – Second Edition (RISB-2) 1992	High school – adulthood[a]	Overall adjustment
Thematic Apperception Test (TAT) 1971	5 years – 79 years	Dominant drives, emotions, conflicts, and complexities of personality
		Perceptions of interpersonal relationships
Roberts Apperception Test for Children: 2 (Roberts-2) 2005	6 years – 18 years	Adaptive and maladaptive or atypical social perceptions
		Scales: Theme overview Available resources Problem identification Resolution Emotion Outcome Unusual or atypical responses
Rorschach Test 2014	5 years – 70 years	Personality structure and dynamics including cognitive, affective-emotional, ego functioning, defenses, conflicts, and coping mechanisms
Structured Interview for Prodromal Syndromes (SIPS) 2001	Adolescence+	Extent of psychosis

Other forms of sentence completion tests can be used with younger children and adolescents proper evidence. Despite this controversy, relatively recent research (e.g., Tibon Czopp & Zeligman, 2016) has demonstrated that the elements of Exner (2009) scoring involving identification of psychotic disorders rest on solid statistical analysis. Accordingly, many clinicians who continue to use the Rorschach (Rorschach, 2014) use it primarily to answer referral questions about an individual's capacity to understand reality in the way that most people understand it.

Finally, contemporary efforts to treat psychosis have reinforced the need for early identification. Early identification allows for implementation of psychiatric, psychotherapeutic, educational, career, and family supports that may forestall full-scale psychosis. To facilitate early identification, test instruments have been designed for administration in the prodromal phase of psychosis (i.e., the period during which symptoms may be suspected or just emerging). Prominent among these instruments is the SIPS (McGlashan et al., 2001). As the name of the test indicates, the SIPS (McGlashan et al., 2001) is completed in a structured interview format and may be used beginning in adolescence. Extensive information is gathered regarding individual and family history, presenting mental health problems, and symptoms indicative of psychosis. Careful interpretation of the test findings indicates whether psychosis seems to be unlikely, approaching, or already established (Table 1).

References

American Psychiatric Association. (2013). *Diagnostic and statistical manual of mental disorders* (5th ed.). American Psychiatric Association.
American Psychological Association Services, Inc. (2014). *About prescribing psychologists.* https://www.apaservices.org/practice/advocacy/authority/prescribing-psychologists.
Burns, R. C., & Kaufman, S. H. (1971). *Kinetic Family Drawings (K-F-D): An Introduction to Understanding Children Through Kinetic Drawings.* Constable.
Cuijpers, P., Sijbrandij, M., Koole, S. L., Andersson, G., Beekman, A. T., & Reynolds, C. F. (2014). Adding psychotherapy to antidepressant medication in depression and anxiety disorders: A meta-analysis. *World Psychiatry, 13*(1), 56–67. https://doi.org/10.1002/wps.20089
Exner, J. E. (2009). *A Rorschach workbook for the comprehensive system.* Rorschach Workshops.
Machover, K. (1949). *Personality projection in the drawing of the human figure: A method of personality investigation.* Charles C. Thomas.
McGlashan, T. H., Miller, T. J., Woods, S. W., Rosen, J. L., Hoffman, R. E., & Davidson, L. (2001). *Structured Interview for Prodromal Syndromes.* PRIME Research Clinic, Yale School of Medicine.
Murray, H. A. (1971). *TAT: Thematic Apperception Test.* Harvard University Press.
Roberts, G. E. (2005). *Roberts Apperception Test for Children: 2.* Psychological Assessment Resources.
Rorschach, H. (2014). *Rorschach Test.* Hogrefe Publishing Group.
Rotter, J. B., Lah, M. I., & Rafferty, J. E. (1992). *RISB-2: Rotter Incomplete Sentences Blank.* (2nd ed.): Psychological Corporation.
Tibon Czopp, S., & Zeligman, R. (2016). The Rorschach comprehensive system (CS) psychometric validity of individual variables. *Journal of Personality Assessment, 98*(4), 335–342. https://doi.org/10.1080/00223891.2015.1131162

Tsuang, M. T., Bar, J. L., Stone, W. S., & Faraone, S. V. (2004). Gene-environment interactions in mental disorders. *World Psychiatry, 3*(2), 73–83.

Uher, R., & Zwicker, A. (2017). Etiology in psychiatry: Embracing the reality of poly-gene-environmental causation of mental illness. *World Psychiatry, 16*(2), 121–129. https://doi.org/10.1002/wps.20436

Developmental Status

Basic Definitions

Developmental status refers to a youngster's developmental progress compared to normative expectations for their age. Abundant research findings allow for specification of when particular developmental milestones typically occur (e.g., Centers for Disease Control and Prevention, 2020). Development is tracked along a variety of critical dimensions. Developmental accomplishments in the cognitive dimension include fundamental identification of objects, recognition of correspondence, evaluation, comparison, prediction, abstraction, and imagination. Developmental accomplishments in the physical dimension include control of body positioning, proficiency in movement, and myriad visual-motor skills. In the interpersonal dimension, developmental accomplishments include eye contact, comfort and pleasure derived from interacting, tolerance for the absence of others, perspective-taking, accommodation to others, and concern for the welfare of others. Finally, in the communication dimension, developmental accomplishments include comprehension and use of facial expressions and gestures, acquisition and use of spoken and written language, and grasp of nuanced elements of communications (e.g., sarcasm).

Why Measure Developmental Status?

Many disorders affecting children and adolescents can be thought of as impairments superimposed on an essentially normal course of development. For example, consider a youngster whose fundamental capacities for communication and interpersonal relatedness are intact and developmentally appropriate, but whose functioning is hampered by crippling social anxiety. On the other hand, disorders that are indistinguishable from a youth's fundamental developmental course are considered

N. E. Moss, L. Moss-Racusin, *Practical Guide to Child and Adolescent Psychological Testing*, Best Practices in Child and Adolescent Behavioral Health Care, https://doi.org/10.1007/978-3-030-73515-9_17

developmental disorders. In such cases, virtually all aspects of functioning display characteristics of the disorder. Autism Spectrum Disorder is the prime example of a developmental disorder. To illustrate, an autistic youth's atypical and excessive physical response to an intrusive peer is itself an expression of the developmental impairments in social communication and regulation that characterize Autism Spectrum Disorder.

Assessment of developmental status has an important role to play with both types of disorders. Firstly, it can clarify which type is occurring for a youngster by allowing for comparison of their development to normative developmental progressions. Secondly, assessment also elucidates a youngster's developmental abilities and impairments in service of facilitating the most appropriate expectations and productive interventions. Above all, the most compelling argument for developmental status assessment is promoting a youth's chance for the best possible ultimate outcomes. The earliest possible intervention in any form of developmental difficulty offers the most hope for a youngster's progress and long-term quality of life. Therefore, assessment of developmental status can and should begin at very young ages for youngsters who exhibit developmental abnormalities (e.g., babies who do not make eye contact).

Common Patterns of Difficulty

Autism Spectrum Disorder

Nature of Difficulty Currently understood as a cluster of related clinical phenomena ranged along a spectrum of specific symptoms and levels of severity, an Autism Spectrum Disorder diagnosis denotes fundamental, inborn, lifelong social impairment. Poor or absent eye contact; idiosyncratic, stereotypic, self-stimulatory behaviors; problematic self-regulation; very poor executive functioning; impulsivity; insufficient adaptive behaviors and prominent maladaptive behaviors; inadequate empathy; disordered social communication; and impaired peer relationships are all characteristic of an Autism Spectrum Disorder.

How Do We Help? As with several of the difficulties discussed earlier, psychoeducation is invaluable for young people on the Autism Spectrum, their families, and all the individuals involved with them. Psychoeducation is particularly useful in regard to Autism Spectrum Disorder, because the social interaction, communication, and behavioral symptoms are easily misunderstood. For example, they are frequently erroneously equated with inferior intelligence, indifference, rudeness, disobedience, and hostility. Furthermore, individuals unfamiliar with Autism Spectrum Disorder are often confused, frightened, or repulsed by those who are on the Spectrum. Accurate, comprehensive psychoeducation can combat such misunderstandings and unfairly negative reactions, in part by prescribing the most useful and practical ways to relate with someone on the Spectrum, thereby increasing clarity, confidence, and acceptance.

A specific form of psychoeducation merits special note. Following a psychological assessment that supports an Autism Spectrum Disorder diagnosis, it is often helpful to convey the findings to relatives beyond those directly involved in the assessment (e.g., parents and caregivers). These relatives can include siblings, grandparents, aunts, uncles, and other extended family members. Hearing from a professional about the diagnosis and receiving information about its causes, treatment, and prognosis often preserve family relationships. Siblings' resentment of caregiver time spent with an autistic youngster, and grandparents' conclusions that their grandchild is spoiled, are examples of the difficulties that can be alleviated through honest, straightforward discussion of an Autism Spectrum Disorder.

Beyond relatives, it is also often very helpful to discuss a youngster's Spectrum diagnosis with their classmates and with all school personnel. Forthright discussion helps destigmatize autistic behavior, instructs schoolmates and school staff in concrete ways to behave with an autistic individual, and generally facilitates more successful interactions in the school setting.

For the affected youngster themselves, psychoeducation can provide a transformative explanation for the poor fit between their ways of functioning and expectations for them from individuals not on the Autism Spectrum. In addition to explanation, psychoeducation may also be able to help an autistic individual begin to learn the meaning of behaviors directed toward them, as well as to convey their thoughts, opinions, and wishes more clearly and acceptably. In so doing, psychoeducation can help decrease self-blame and increase self-esteem.

Youngsters on the Autism Spectrum can also benefit from a host of school-based interventions. Critical among these is special education. Federal and state laws prescribe the procedure by which families and school districts can collaborate to produce an Individualized Educational Plan in order to meet the particular educational needs of a student (Volkmar & Wiesner, 2017). The Individualized Educational Plan specifies the subject areas in which specialized academic instruction is necessary, along with the instructional and environmental accommodations needed for the student's education. Academic progress is monitored continuously and reevaluated at legally mandated intervals, thus allowing for modifications to Individualized Educational Plans in order to maximize gains. As students get older, special education also includes legally prescribed preparation for transition to young adulthood. (Please find additional information about the special education process in the Types of Psychological Assessments and the School Psychoeducational Assessment Process chapters.)

Additional school-based interventions include school-based mental health services (described in the Social-Emotional Functioning chapter), peer mentoring programs, and specific jobs within the school (e.g., bringing items to the main office), all with the aim of more fully integrating students with an Autism Spectrum Disorder. Treatments such as speech-language therapy (e.g., to facilitate intelligible speech production, as well as higher order grasp and usage of language for communication), physical therapy (e.g., to improve balance, coordination, and body control), and occupational therapy (e.g., to enhance sensory processing, motor planning, and performance of specific motor actions) can also be provided in the school setting if a youngster's deficits in these areas have a demonstrable negative effect on their educational progress and functioning in the school environment. If the deficits do not hinder adequate educational progress and functioning, these treatments can be pursued outside of the school setting.

Youth with an Autism Spectrum Disorder can also benefit from a range of other mental health services (again as described in the Social-Emotional Functioning chapter). To provide examples of how these services can relate specifically to the Autism Spectrum, individual therapy can help a youngster on the Spectrum tackle anxiety related to daily peer interactions. Parent and caregiver counseling can improve adult responses to the needs of youngsters with an Autism Spectrum Disorder (e.g., to sleep on the floor under their bed rather than in it). Family therapy can assist families in their efforts to preserve their personal relationships in the face of demands and difficulties related to a youngster's Autism Spectrum Disorder. Social skills groups – a type of educational group therapy mentioned in the Social-Emotional Functioning chapter – are very useful for youngsters who struggle with reading social cues, managing social communication, initiating and responding to peer interactions, and maintaining the self-regulation necessary for productive inter-personal relationships. Through structured social activity and thorough guidance from trained therapists, youngsters learn, practice, and refine interpersonal skills that facilitate acceptance and pleasure with peers.

For mental health services to be useful for individuals on the Autism Spectrum, it is critical that the professionals involved have special training and expertise related to Spectrum disorders. Without it, the professionals risk profound misunder-standing of autistic symptomatology. One common misunderstanding is attributing an autistic individual's overt distress to complex, deeply rooted inner turmoil rather than to panic over a failure to grasp the social demands of a current situation. The radically different interventions that result from each of these interpretations under-line the need for special Autism Spectrum training, which increases the likelihood of accurate interpretations and effective interventions.

Many community-based activities can also be beneficial to youngsters with an Autism Spectrum Disorder. Some of them are designed specifically for people on the Spectrum, while others are directed toward the population at large. The key fac-tor for determining if an activity will be appropriate and pleasant for a youngster on the Spectrum is the group leader's ability to understand and accommodate an autis-tic individual's needs. Typically useful community activities include martial arts classes, swimming lessons, therapeutic horseback riding, faith-based youth groups, scouting, art endeavors, and participation in theater productions. Each of these activities has the potential to provide knowledge, satisfaction, and socialization to an autistic youngster.

Prominent Instruments

Again, psychological assessment of developmental status has the greatest potential to enhance quality of life when performed as early as possible. Early assessment allows for intervention that can forestall or even prevent consolidation of less than optimal developmental functioning.

Assessment of developmental status is approached in two main ways. The first is used when concern is raised about an infant or toddler's acquisition of skills. In these situations, direct assessment is carried out in a formal testing setting, usually with the support of a parent or caregiver. To maximize the child's comfort and performance, procedures are designed to mimic interactive play experiences. Engagement in these experiences makes it possible to determine how on pace the child's early verbal, visual-spatial, motor, and interactive abilities are with those of their age-mates. As an example, playful building and knocking down of a block tower allows for assessment of the child's early fine motor coordination.

The second type of developmental status assessment occurs when specific concern is raised about a youngster having an identifiable developmental disorder. Youngsters participating in this kind of assessment complete behavior checklists and attempt to interact with a psychologist in prescribed ways. For example, youngsters may be presented with diverse play materials, such as a plastic dinosaur, a feather, and a small paper umbrella, and instructed to make up and enact a narrative. Such a task assesses perspective-taking and hypothetical thinking in order to inform a potential diagnosis of an Autism Spectrum Disorder. In addition, respondents familiar with the youngsters contribute their observations by also completing checklists and sharing pertinent anecdotal information.

The Bayley Scales of Infant and Toddler Development (Bayley-4; Bayley & Aylward, 2019) and the Mullen Scales of Early Learning (Mullen, 1995) are two primary instruments used to track development in the earliest months and years of life. While the tests differ somewhat on organization and labeling of developmental domains, they both use a structured, play-based, interactive format to examine emergence of communication skills, maturation of motor skills, and interpersonal progress. They tend to be used to follow the aftereffects of known illness or injury at birth or during infancy. They are also used when early development proceeds in an unexpected, inappropriate direction without a known cause. Results on these tests can help assess the potential clinical significance of any deviation from typical developmental pathways.

The Autism Diagnostic Observation Schedule (ADOS-2; Lord et al., 2012), the Social Responsiveness Scale (SRS-2; Constantino & Gruber, 2012), and the Childhood Autism Rating Scale (CARS2; Schopler, 2010) are more specialized instruments used in the assessment and diagnosis of Autism Spectrum Disorder. The ADOS-2 (Lord et al., 2012) is a highly structured, interactive observation of a youngster's capacities for flexible thinking, interpersonal relatedness, emotional expression, and verbal and nonverbal communication. It yields a combination of qualitative ratings and quantitative scores. The SRS-2 (Constantino & Gruber, 2012) and CARS2 (Schopler, 2010) are both checklists that focus directly on the presence or absence of specific symptoms of Autism Spectrum Disorder. Both of these tests provide quantitative scores (Table 1).

Table 1 Prominent instruments for assessing developmental status

Test name and publication date	Age range	Information provided by test
Bayley Scales of Infant and Toddler Development – Fourth Edition (Bayley-4) 2019	16 days – 42 months	Cognitive Language Motor Social-emotional Adaptive behavior
Mullen Scales of Early Learning 1995	Birth – 68 months	Gross motor Visual reception Fine motor Expressive language Receptive language
Autism Diagnostic Observation Schedule – Second Edition (ADOS-2) 2012	12 months – adulthood	Communication Social interaction Play Restricted and repetitive behaviors
Social Responsiveness Scale – Second Edition (SRS-2) 2012	2 years, 6 months – adulthood	Social awareness Social cognition Social communication Social motivation Restricted interests and repetitive behaviors
Childhood Autism Rating Scale – Second Edition (CARS2) 2010	2+ years	Relating to people Imitation Social-emotional Understanding Emotional response Emotional expression and regulation of emotions Body use Object use Object use in play Adaptation to change Restricted interests Visual response Listening response Taste/smell/touch response and use Fear or nervousness Fear or anxiety Verbal communication Nonverbal communication Activity level Thinking/cognitive integration skills Level and consistency of intellectual response General impressions

References

Bayley, N., & Aylward, G. (2019). *Bayley Scales of Infant and Toddler Development* (4th ed.). NCS Pearson.

Centers for Disease Control and Prevention. (2020). *CDC's developmental milestones.* https://www.cdc.gov/ncbddd/actearly/milestones/index.html

Constantino, J. N., & Gruber, C. P. (2012). *SRS-2: Social Responsiveness Scale.* Western Psychological Services.

Lord, C., DiLavore, P. C., Gotham, K., Guthrie, W., Luyster, R. J., Risi, S., & Rutter, M. (2012). *ADOS-2: Autism Diagnostic Observation Schedule* (2nd ed.). Western Psychological Services.

Mullen, E. (1995). *Mullen Scales of Early Learning.* NCS Pearson.

Schopler, E. (2010). *CARS2: Childhood Autism Rating Scale.* Western Psychological Services.

Volkmar, F. R., & Wiesner, L. A. (2017). *Essential clinical guide to understanding and treating autism.* Wiley.

Conclusion

Primary care providers of children and adolescents are continually challenged to understand, explain, and relieve a wide array of difficulties in their patients. Despite thorough training and valuable expertise, providers often need additional information when they encounter youth who present with psychological, behavioral, and educational problems that defy easy solutions. Psychological testing provides just such additional information.

By crafting clear, specific referral questions and directing them, if possible, to a psychologist with whom a productive, collegial relationship has been established, a primary care provider can prompt the assessment process. Difficult individual characteristics, family issues, school struggles, a requirement to prove eligibility for specialized programming, and the need to facilitate progress in an otherwise stalled treatment are all appropriate focus points for psychological testing.

With some variation related to setting and specific type of testing, the assessment itself progresses through identifiable stages. These stages are gathering a history; carrying out naturalistic observations, as appropriate; getting input from all relevant sources; conducting the face-to-face assessment sessions; providing feedback to those most involved with the youngster and with the youngster themselves; generating a written report; and following up, as indicated. Depending on the particular referral questions, the assessment can investigate many domains of functioning. These include intelligence, speech-language competence, visual-motor coordination, memory operation, attention and concentration, executive functioning, academic achievement, overall behavior, adaptive functioning, social-emotional condition, and developmental status.

Just as the primary care provider may be the one to prompt the assessment, so too may they lead implementation of the assessment findings and recommendations once the testing is completed. Through careful reading and interpretation of each section in the written report, the primary care provider can formulate an individualized, fully informed treatment plan.

© Springer Nature Switzerland AG 2021

N. E. Moss, L. Moss-Racusin, *Practical Guide to Child and Adolescent Psychological Testing*, Best Practices in Child and Adolescent Behavioral Health Care, https://doi.org/10.1007/978-3-030-73515-9_18

As noted throughout this book, all consumers of psychological test reports are urged to make active, ongoing use of the information provided. A report that is filed away and ignored is a symbol of a failed psychological assessment and a lost opportunity for a youngster. In contrast, a report that serves repeatedly as a reference point and guide for psychological, educational, and medical efforts represents the sort of collaborative endeavor that best enhances a youngster's continued wellbeing and progress.

Psychological Assessment Report Example

Name: Haley Smith
Assessment Dates: 09/29/2020, 10/05/2020, 10/12/2020, 10/16/2020, 10/27/2020,
   11/04/2020
Birthdate: 11-28-06
School: Lupine Middle School
Age: 13 years
Grade: 8
Haley identifies as White and female.

Identifying Information Annotation

This section provides a very brief foundation of demographic information. This information anchors the data to follow, specifically in relation to chronological time, the patient's age, and their academic grade level.

When identifying information sections reveal a high number of testing sessions (i.e., more than four to six), the reader can see that there was some difficulty with timely assessment completion. Most often, such delay reflects a youngster's slow work pace, but it may also reflect caregiver difficulties participating in the assessment (e.g., missing appointments due to work obligations).

When there is a lack of typical correspondence between a youngster's age and grade level, the youngster likely experienced retentions earlier in schooling, advancements in academic standing, and/or lengthy interruptions in school attendance. These events and their explanations should be documented in the report.

© Springer Nature Switzerland AG 2021   133
N. E. Moss, L. Moss-Racusin, *Practical Guide to Child and Adolescent*
Psychological Testing, Best Practices in Child and Adolescent Behavioral
Health Care, https://doi.org/10.1007/978-3-030-73515-9_19

Background and Referral

Ms. Smith, Haley's mother, provided background information for the current assessment. Maternal report indicated that Haley was the product of a planned pregnancy. The pregnancy was remarkable for Ms. Smith's significant weight gain and periodic bleeding, evidently due to uterine cysts. The bleeding necessitated a couple of emergency room visits, but the pregnancy remained viable. Haley was delivered by a planned Cesarean procedure, all cysts were removed, and both Haley and her mother were considered to be in good health.

Ms. Smith described Haley as an "easy newborn." The family co-slept, and Haley slept well from the beginning of her life. Haley was breast-fed until the age of four years. If upset, she could be soothed. Ms. Smith believed that Haley reached all early developmental milestones in a timely manner. Ms. Smith stated, though, that she suspected that Haley might have an Autism Spectrum Disorder. Her suspicion grew out of observations of Haley's poor eye contact and rigid, repetitive play.

In terms of her personal medical history, Haley had a serious allergic reaction to lentil soup at the age of five years. She had trouble breathing and was treated in the emergency room. Based on that experience, Haley was diagnosed with a legume allergy. Haley was also seen in the emergency room once for a severe, flu-type virus. In terms of extended family medical status, among Haley's blood relatives there was a history of Learning Disorders; severe mental illness including Bipolar Disorder, depression, and self-injurious behavior; excessive use of alcohol; and possible eating disorder.

Haley's earliest care was provided by her mother. When Ms. Smith had to return to work approximately three months after Haley's birth, Mr. Smith, Haley's father, became Haley's primary caregiver under the close guidance and supervision of Ms. Smith. Sadly, when Haley was almost three years old, her parents separated, and her father ceased all contact with Haley and her mother. Ms. Smith assumed all parenting responsibilities from that time forward.

Haley successfully attended a private preschool in a nearby town. For kindergarten, she transitioned into her local public school system. At the first grade level, she encountered marked difficulty at school. Based on a teacher's referral, Haley was evaluated and found to qualify for special education. Receiving multidisciplinary services, Haley remained a special education student until the fifth grade. At that point, although there was consensus that Haley likely had an Autism Spectrum Disorder, she was believed to be doing well enough to be exited from special education. She encountered more difficulty in the sixth grade and was served through a 504 Plan through the seventh grade. During these years, Ms. Smith spent many hours at home supplementing Haley's academic instruction. Haley herself spent many more hours than her teachers required to complete her homework. At times, she even did more work than was assigned. Ms. Smith described this work at home as quite burdensome.

During the second half of her seventh grade year, Haley became extremely distressed over a misunderstood social encounter in the school setting. She seemed completely unaware of the inappropriateness of her own behavior. Due to lack of awareness, she continued to display unacceptable behavior despite many adult efforts to redirect her. Ms. Smith asserted that Haley was just trying to "be entertaining." She believed that Haley's behavior was a misguided attempt to socialize. Regardless, Haley was suspended for one week.

Following that suspension, both outpatient and school-based evaluations were carried out. Haley's Autism Spectrum Disorder diagnosis was confirmed, and multidisciplinary services were recommended. Haley reentered special education as an eighth grade student. However, there was then a disagreement between Ms. Smith and her advocate, Ms. Crowley, on one side, and school personnel, on the other side. The disagreement centered on the adequacy of Haley's Individualized Educational Plan. Ms. Smith and Ms. Crowley asserted that Haley's weaknesses and needs were far greater than the school district appreciated. School district personnel stated that Haley had substantial competence in the school setting.

To address these different appraisals of Haley's level of functioning, it was agreed upon to pursue an independent educational evaluation. The public school Director of Student Services referred Haley for the current assessment. To direct the assessment, the Planning and Placement Team generated the following specific referral questions:

1. *Adaptive behaviors at home versus school? The Team sees Haley as capable of problem-solving and of completing tasks independently.*
2. *Work completion at home versus school? The Team sees Haley able to complete tasks in a timely fashion at school. Ms. Smith is telling us that Haley is spending five hours a night on homework. How can there be such discrepancy? A homework chart has been used to document time spent completing homework. The chart has encouraged Haley to stick to a timeline for each subject.*

Background and Referral Annotation

As discussed earlier, the aim of this section of a report is to focus on aspects of a youngster's early developmental course, personal and familial medical history, and educational progress that pertain to the referral questions that prompted the assessment. The section concludes with a clear statement of the referral source and questions.

For this example case, several early developmental features are noteworthy. Haley had prenatal vulnerability due to a problematic pregnancy (i.e., maternal bleeding). While such bleeding does not inevitably lead to later disorders, it does suggest the possibility of a weakened developmental foundation that could lead to further difficulty across the life span. It was also notable that Haley was breast-fed for a longer period of time than most infants in the United States (Centers for Disease Control and Prevention, 2020). Again, such a feeding pattern is not necessarily cause for concern, and could simply reflect family preference. However, it might signify some difficulty with moving on toward independent eating. The reader should keep these aspects of Haley's history in mind but suspend diagnostic conclusions until reading further data.

In relation to medical health, the reader should take note of Haley's allergy and need for hospital visits. Likewise, the reader should register the significance of Haley's family's medical and psychological history. The family history of Learning Disorders and severe mental illness are likely particularly relevant to Haley's diagnostic status. The unfortunate departure of Haley's father is also significant. Information about his abandonment and about the subsequent required shifts in parenting of Haley should alert the reader to consider the impact of trauma on Haley's overall development and wellbeing.

This section of the report also traces the course of Haley's Autism Spectrum Disorder diagnosis. The reader should note when concerns were first raised by one parent and how those worries were later addressed by educational and healthcare professionals. Like many individuals on the Autism Spectrum, Haley had to weather being understood in different ways at different points in time. These differences in diagnostic appraisal led to premature suspension of special services to Haley. Fortunately, Haley was ultimately returned to special education, but not before a particular disruptive incident, characteristic of youngsters on the Autism Spectrum, occurred. The reader should understand the description of this incident as support for Haley's diagnosis.

It is important to note that Haley has several reported strengths. She reached most early developmental milestones within a typical timeframe, she could be soothed as an infant, her preschool and kindergarten experiences were successful, and some of her academic achievements were on par with her agemates. This information can reassure the reader that, although Haley has a serious diagnosis, she still has the capacity for meaningful progress.

The section concludes with a description of the ongoing disagreement between Haley's mother and school district. This description leads into the nature of the referral for the current assessment. Rather than focus on fundamental diagnostic questions, the current assessment aims to resolve conflict regarding the manifestation of a known diagnosis, as well as to provide guidance about how best to serve Haley in the context of conflict resolution.

Assessment Instruments

Review of previous evaluations
School observation
Meeting with educators
Behavioral observations in assessment setting
Kaufman Assessment Battery for Children – Second Edition Normative Update (KABC-II NU)
Wechsler Intelligence Scale for Children – Fifth Edition (WISC V)

Working Memory and Processing Speed Domains; Cognitive Proficiency
Behavior Rating Inventory of Executive Function, Second Edition (BRIEF2)

   Self-report form
NEPSY – Second Edition (NEPSY-II)

   Auditory Attention and Response Set, Comprehension of Instructions, and
   Narrative Memory subtests
Beery-Buktenica Developmental Test of Visual-Motor Integration – Sixth Edition
   (BEERY VMI)
Kaufman Test of Educational Achievement – Third Edition (KTEA-3)

   Form B
Behavior Assessment System for Children – Third Edition (BASC-3)

   Self-report form
Machover Draw-A-Person Test (DAP)
Kinetic Family Drawing (KFD)
Rotter Incomplete Sentences Blank – Second Edition (RISB-2)

Assessment Instruments Annotation

The assessment procedures and instruments are presented so that the reader may know the sources of the psychologist's conclusions. It is important for the reader to be alert to test editions and forms so as to ensure that up-to-date, appropriate measures were used, and that conclusions can be considered valid. The procedures and instruments are listed in conceptual order (i.e., the order in which the data are presented). This sort of ordering minimizes the cognitive organization required of readers, thereby making it easier for them to follow the information provided.

Review of Previous Evaluations

Date	Type of Evaluation	Main Findings	Main Recommendations
March, 2014	Speech-Language Evaluation	Speech-Language: Receptive, expressive, and pragmatic language within normal limits. Poor speech intelligibility.	Speech-Language: Weekly speech-language therapy for 12 weeks.
		Diagnosis: Phonological disorder diagnosed.	

(Continued)

Date	Type of Evaluation	Main Findings	Main Recommendations
November, 2015	Psychoeducational Evaluation	*Intelligence:* Borderline, inconsistent intelligence. Weakness in working memory and processing speed.	*Educational:* Specific teaching strategies.
		Academic Achievement: Average/Below average academic achievement.	*Assessment:* Further language testing.
		Social: Generally average social skills but somewhat limited assertiveness and cooperation.	
		Behavioral: Behavioral difficulties mainly involving unusual social behaviors, interpersonal withdrawal, and poor functional communication.	
November, 2015	Speech-Language Evaluation	*Speech-Language:* Weaknesses in auditory comprehension, higher level problem-solving, and pragmatic language.	*Speech-Language:* Speech-language therapy to improve comprehension, social language, and problem-solving.
		Behavioral: "Spacing out" and unusual behaviors noted during testing.	
November, 2015	Physical Therapy Evaluation	*Motor:* Evaluation focused on gross motor skills. Locomotor skills adequate, but deficiency in object control skills, and immature coordination noted.	*Motor:* Two years of school-based physical therapy.
November, 2015	Occupational Therapy Evaluation	*Social:* Social impairments noted.	*Motor:* Occupational therapy to focus on visual-motor and visual-perceptual development.
		Motor: Adequate visual-perceptual skills but impaired visual-motor coordination. Immature grasp and poor handwriting.	
		Sensory: Mild sensory problems related to attentional difficulty.	

(Continued)

Date	Type of Evaluation	Main Findings	Main Recommendations
October, 2018	Educational Evaluation	Academic Achievement: Slightly uneven but largely average academic achievements.	Educational: Extended time on class written assignments, quizzes, and tests.
October, 2018	Psychoeducational Evaluation	Intelligence: Low average intelligence. Working memory and processing speed better than in 2013; difference not explained.	Educational: Engage in educational activities.
		Diagnosis: Teacher ratings argued against an Autism Spectrum Disorder diagnosis, except for the ratings of special education teacher, which were indicative of problematic social skills and an Autism Spectrum Disorder diagnosis. Maternal ratings argued that an Autism Spectrum Disorder diagnosis was very likely correct. Examiner concluded that Haley presented differently in the home versus school environments.	Speech-Language: Develop vocabulary.
			Behavioral: Keep a daily schedule/routine. State clear expectations.
			Assessment: Integrate multidisciplinary findings.
November, 2018	Speech-Language Evaluation	Speech-Language: Language scores ranged from marginal to average. Understanding of semantic relationships and grasping orally conveyed information were particular weaknesses. Still, overall improvement from previous assessment.	Speech-Language: Continue services.

(Continued)

Date	Type of Evaluation	Main Findings	Main Recommendations
May, 2020	Psychological Evaluation	Intelligence: Modestly average intelligence.	Educational: Designation as a special education student in the Autism category. Specialized academic instruction. Help with organization and time management. Any indicated educationally-needed therapies.
		Behavioral: Well below average adaptive behavior. Significant behavioral distress associated with social and academic problems, separation fears, and perfectionistic/compulsive behaviors.	
		Motor: Low average visual-motor coordination.	
		Diagnosis: Further test results confirmed Autism Spectrum Disorder diagnosis. Haley was seen as ranking in the severe range.	Speech-Language: Renewed weekly home-based speech-language therapy.
			Psychological: Continued home-based psychotherapy.
			Social: Weekly school-based group social skills training.
			Behavioral: Home-based Applied Behavior Analysis services.
			Assessment: Further school-based speech-language and occupational therapy evaluations. Home-based reassessment two years in the future.
June, 2020	Speech-Language Evaluation	Speech-Language: Modestly average single word receptive and expressive vocabularies. Below average comprehension of broader spoken language. Uneven below average curriculum-relevant language and literacy skills. Below average pragmatic language and clear social communication deficits.	Speech-Language: Speech-language therapy to promote understanding of metaphors, idioms, and conversational skills.
		Diagnosis: Social-Pragmatic Language disorder, moderate-severe.	Assessment: Share findings at Planning and Placement Team meeting.

(Continued)

Date	Type of Evaluation	Main Findings	Main Recommendations
June, 2020	Occupational Therapy Evaluation	Behavioral: Teacher ratings indicated below average overall adaptive behavior skills. More specifically, communication was below average, daily living skills were modestly average, and socialization was below average.	Educational: Check work for understanding. Ask Haley to repeat instructions or use visual aids to ensure understanding. Use of nonverbal cueing to enhance Haley's classroom engagement. Continued academic support for organization. Continued parent-teacher communication.
		Executive Functioning: Marked problems with executive functioning noted in home environment but not school environment.	Assessment: Parental sharing of present assessment findings with the pediatrician and other involved professionals. Share findings at Planning and Placement Team meeting.

Review of Previous Evaluations Annotation

For Haley, this report section is lengthy, since she had completed numerous evaluations prior to the current assessment. It is important to note that in a real report, the names and credentials of the examiners would be documented for each evaluation. The reader should take particular note of Haley's long involvement with special education and mental health professionals, as well as of the documentation of her modest cognitive abilities. Wrestling with the Autism Spectrum Diagnosis and struggles over the appropriate amount and type of special education should be understood as the most important threads in these summarized evaluation findings.

School Observation

Haley was observed in two classes at her middle school. The first portion of the observation took place in her math class. As instructed, the students arranged their desks into groupings of four. Haley, however, situated her desk at an odd angle to only one other student. Under the teacher's direction, the class went over a previous difficult homework assignment and then moved on to a lesson on factors. Haley sat quietly throughout the review and lesson. It was impossible to infer her level of understanding. The teacher continued giving information, expecting the students to take notes. Haley did so but less extensively than her peers. The class was then told to solve a problem on their own. Haley began to work only when the teacher went over to prompt and help her. Homework was then distributed, and 15 minutes were provided for the students to make a start on the assignment. Haley remained quietly immobile. She then raised her hand for help, and the teacher returned to her, but by then, the class was being dismissed.

There was considerable peer interaction in Haley's math class. When allowed, the students socialized quietly. They also worked collaboratively to a great extent. Haley, however, was entirely removed from this interaction. She remained uninvolved in all conversation. Even the student who was sitting closest to her reached out to other students for help, rather than talking to Haley. Haley's only acknowledgement of others was a silent smile when she overheard a couple of jokes between the teacher and another student.

The second portion of the observation took place in Haley's gym class. The entire class was engaged in a very active, complicated, lengthy relay race. Haley participated as instructed, but her running seemed slightly uncoordinated, and she tired relatively quickly. Again, she engaged in the absolute minimum of peer interaction. When the period ended, Haley ran out of the gym.

Overall, it was clear that Haley is a quiet, well-behaved, cooperative student. At the same time, it was equally clear that she is essentially alone, even when surrounded by many other people. She seems to lack the necessary skill to take social initiative. The absence of overtures by her peers also suggested strongly that, instead of seeing Haley as a potential companion, they are accustomed to her isolation.

School Observation Annotation

The reader should draw two main conclusions from this section of the report. The first is that Haley received attention from her teachers related to class activities, and that with individualized prompts, encouragements, and demonstrations, she was able to participate in mainstream educational instruction. This conclusion is optimistic and encouraging for Haley. The second conclusion is that Haley's essential isolation, including while physically surrounded by others, was going unnoticed and/or unaddressed by the teachers. Acknowledgement of the absence of connection between Haley and her peers was critical for understanding her situation and for planning the most useful programming for her as she approached high school.

Although it could be tempting to fault Haley's instructors for failing to notice or address her isolation, it would be unfair to attribute their lack of acknowledgement to negative intent. Teachers have the weighty responsibility of managing many kinds of behavior while also imparting knowledge to large numbers of students. It can be difficult to register, let alone address, each student's experience at all times. Often, teachers scan a group of students in a classroom or gym, observe that the group as a whole is doing well, and move on to their next responsibility. Many times, a single student's difficulty is readily visible only to an outside observer who is not also charged with academic endeavors and management of a full class.

Summary of Meeting with Educators

Right after the classroom observations, a group discussion was held to gather more information, perceptions, and concerns regarding Haley's educational progress. The instructional disciplines and specialized services represented were language arts, social studies, math, science, learning support, and speech-language.

Haley's language arts teacher stated that Haley was a member of a 14-student class. He described the class as an inclusive, kind group of youngsters who accepted Haley despite her social awkwardness. The teacher attributed this peer acceptance to the students having grown up with Haley. The teacher's report indicated that Haley was a diligent, conscientious student who participated well in book discussions and competently completed reading and writing assignments.

Haley's social studies teacher indicated that Haley's class was quite large but that she was doing well in it. The teacher said that Haley could work independently and engage in appropriate self-advocacy. She stated further that Haley raised appropriate questions to clarify her understanding of relevant material. She also commented, though, on Haley's marked social awkwardness and inability to grasp jokes enjoyed by her classmates. Despite her awkwardness, the teacher stated that Haley's peers treated her well.

Haley's math teacher stated that Haley was in a fast-paced math class. Due to the advanced level of the class, Haley was earning somewhat lower grades. Nevertheless, Haley asked good questions and got help from the teacher, as needed. The teacher recommended that Haley stay at this same class level and re-take the subject as a high school first year. She believed that Haley's prior familiarity with the material would help Haley as a ninth grade math student. The teacher also said that Haley did more work in class and at home than was necessary.

Haley's science teacher described her as a conscientious, independent student. She stated that Haley asked questions when necessary and engaged in good peer interactions. The teacher noted that Haley did better during the second term than during the first term. She "held her own" with class material but struggled more with quizzes. She had the opportunity to re-take the quizzes, though. The teacher also allowed Haley extra time to complete her work. The teacher highlighted two particular difficulties. First, Haley sometimes rejected help from the teacher and from her learning support teachers, seeming to have a poor reaction to constructive criticism. Second, at times, Haley was disorganized. For example, she would bring many unnecessary materials from her locker to class but forget her science notebook.

One of Haley's learning support teachers said that Haley always waited for her, wanting to check and re-check her work. At times, she was not actually in need of academic help but rather needed clarification of assignments and expectations along with reassurance. The teacher helped Haley plan her daily homework to guard against spending too much time working at home. She also helped Haley with organization of materials.

The speech-language specialist had long familiarity with Haley. She recalled that, as a kindergarten student, Haley had made good eye contact. At the time of the current assessment, the specialist saw Haley in a social communication group. In the group, Haley reportedly would become anxious when she was with more unfamiliar peers. Also, while quiet when less knowledgeable about a topic, Haley could participate well in conversation and make appropriate incidental comments. The specialist stated that while Haley had clear skills, she did appear socially awkward. The specialist expressed that Haley's awkwardness might have reflected her introversion, as well as diagnostic characteristics.

Overall, the educators indicated that they understand Haley to be a reasonably competent student, who is able to make good eye contact and interact with others. At the same time, they acknowledged that she works at a somewhat slow pace and that her social connections are relatively superficial. They also recognized the contrast between home-based and school-based appraisals of Haley's competence. Additionally, educators described Haley as overly precise and perfectionistic. They are concerned by her excessive worry about homework and by her burdening herself with work, even when it is not assigned. The educators seem to view Haley's difficulties and concerning behaviors as distinct characteristics unrelated to her Autism Spectrum Disorder diagnosis.

Summary of Meeting with Educators Annotation

This portion of the report summarized a conference with Haley's educators. They presented a consistent portrayal of Haley as a reasonably competent student, who sometimes needed help with efficiency, organization, following directions, and resisting the pull to do more than was required. They also recognized that Haley displayed some social awkwardness. These observations were accurate and helpful.

Discouragingly, however, the educators seemed to downplay the significance of Haley's Autism Spectrum Disorder and its role in the struggles they described her having. Since Haley could meet prescribed demands in the school setting, the educators seemed to minimize the interference of her disorder in home-based and broader interpersonal functioning. Relatedly, they also did not seem to recognize the extent of her social isolation. In keeping with federal law that holds public school districts responsible for providing the most appropriate and comprehensive educational plan for individuals with special needs, the reader should expect the recommendations section of this report to put forth strategies designed to more fully address the manifestations of Haley's disorder across settings.

Behavioral Observations in Assessment Setting

Haley presented as a neatly attired adolescent. Somewhat remarkably, she often wore a red, white, and blue, sequined vest. When asked if this unusual clothing had any special significance to her, Haley replied that she "just liked it." Haley's presentation was also remarkable for the plastic rocket ship that she brought to each testing session. Except for the moments when testing required the use of both hands,

Haley manipulated this figure throughout the assessment. Again, when asked, Haley stated that she "just liked it" and felt good when she could hold the figure. Haley seemed to remain unaware of the atypicality of these aspects of her presentation.

In regard to the assessment tasks, Haley was quietly and consistently cooperative. She did work very slowly, though. Much more than the typical amount of time was needed to complete several of the test instruments. Moreover, there were manifestations, even in the assessment setting, of Haley's belief that she has to do more than is actually expected of her. The clearest example of this vulnerability involved completion of the Beery-Buktenica Developmental Test of Visual-Motor Integration (BEERY VMI), a measure of visual-motor coordination. This test consists of a booklet containing printed representations of increasingly complicated geometric forms. The nature of the printing is such that the lines comprising the forms have tiny but visible widths. They can be perceived as rectangles by overly-conscientious individuals, but they are intended to be understood as single lines. Consistent with standard procedure, Haley was instructed to copy each form as exactly as possible. The first few shapes are quite simple (i.e., vertical and horizontal lines). Like many youngsters, Haley at first took great care to draw perfect, small-dimension rectangles to duplicate the lines in the test booklet. The psychologist then told Haley that single lines would be entirely satisfactory and reassured her that the effort to make perfectly proportioned rectangles was unnecessary. Unlike most youngsters, though, Haley could not accept this reassurance. She continued making perfect, time-intensive rectangles until the designs were simply too complex to allow for her approach.

Haley had to clarify assessment instructions often. In some instances, the same instructions had to be verified more than once. These clarifications and verifications did not seem attributable to Haley being distracted, but rather to her being intent on reassuring herself that she was doing just what was asked of her. She seemed to distrust her perception and grasp of the instructions. In the assessment setting, it was relatively easy for the psychologist to help Haley move on, despite her tendencies to re-check directions and to work excessively. In more real life settings, though, particularly when tackling homework, Haley's difficulties with correct assessment of workload and accurate grasp of instructions would presumably become much more intrusive and burdensome.

Overall, Haley put forth excellent effort on every aspect of the assessment. Given Haley's diligence, the findings reported below should be understood as an accurate representation of her current functioning.

Behavioral Observations in Assessment Setting Annotation

This section of the report provides a foundation for interpreting the remaining test results. The descriptions of Haley support the Autism Spectrum Disorder diagnosis by providing evidence of her idiosyncrasy. The descriptions also highlight that her slow work pace, perfectionism, inability to restrict herself to the actual required work, poor grasp of instructions, and struggle to move on without adult support – all of which had been described by other observers – manifested in the current assessment setting, as well. These pervasive tendencies of Haley's reflect problems with executive functioning, which are consistent with her Autism Spectrum Disorder. The main point of this section for the reader, though, is that Haley worked well enough on assessment tasks for the data to be deemed trustworthy and useful.

Assessment Findings

Haley's intelligence was examined using the Second Edition Normative Update of the Kaufman Assessment Battery for Children (KABC-II NU). The KABC-II NU is derived from neuropsychological research and defines intelligence as mental processing or problem-solving ability. As measured by the KABC-II NU, Haley placed relatively low in the below average range of overall intellectual ability. However, her Fluid-Crystallized Intelligence Index, an Intelligence Quotient equivalent, should be interpreted cautiously, since there was significant variability within and across cognitive domains.

The Sequential Processing Domain measures step-by-step, linear problem-solving. Due to the significant discrepancy between Haley's subtest scores in this domain, her below average overall domain score is less meaningful. It is more useful to directly examine the subtest scores. Haley earned an average score on Number Recall, a subtest that required her to listen to and then repeat increasingly long strings of numbers. This is a relatively rote task, on which she performed adequately. In contrast, Word Order is a much more complex task, requiring the coordination of auditory, visual, and kinesthetic information. This complexity was more than Haley could manage, and she earned a markedly deficient score on this subtest. Thus, it should be concluded that Haley has adequate sequential processing for relatively simple tasks.

The Simultaneous Processing Domain investigates more holistic, integrative problem-solving. In this domain, Haley's performance was much more consistent and ranked in the below average range.

The Planning Domain examines higher order mental organization. Somewhat surprisingly, Haley placed consistently in the average range in this domain. On Story Completion, she was able to correctly arrange pictures that laid out simple stories. On Pattern Reasoning, she was able to infer nonverbal, conceptual relationships between pictures of objects and forms. In all likelihood, Haley did relatively well on these tasks, because they were highly structured and offered a limited number of choices to arrive at a correct response. She was free from the need to structure or limit the tasks herself.

The Learning and Knowledge Domains are measures of how well Haley takes in new information. The Learning Domain assessed Haley's competence with immediate recall of novel information. Her performance in this domain was consistently below average. In contrast, the Knowledge Domain assessed Haley's competence at deriving information from her environment over time. Her overall Knowledge Domain score is less meaningful, because of the discrepancy between her subtest scores. On Verbal Knowledge, Haley placed in the average range, displaying an adequate fund of general, factual information. On Riddles, though, Haley placed in the deficient range. This subtest presented Haley with several segments of information but required her to organize the information and produce a response without any identified options from which to choose. This task was quite difficult for Haley.

Overall, then, as measured by the KABC-II NU, Haley has uneven but generally below average intelligence. It is striking to compare her KABC-II NU performance with her performance on an alternative intelligence test administered in May, 2020. As part of the earlier assessment, Haley earned an Intelligence Quotient estimated to be in the modestly average range. This score was based on only two subtests, though, and both of them capitalized on Haley's relative strengths (i.e., ability to make use of structure and a limited number of response choices, along with general verbal knowledge). As a more comprehensive measure, the KABC-II NU should be seen as a more valid indicator of Haley's broad cognitive functioning (Table 1).

To address parental and educator reports of Haley needing inordinate amounts of time to finish homework, the Working Memory and Processing Speed subtests on the Fifth Edition of the Wechsler Intelligence Scale for Children (WISC V) were administered. Administration of these domains also allowed for derivation of an overall Cognitive Proficiency score.

Working memory is the capacity to keep necessary information in mind while carrying out associated cognitive tasks. As shown below, Haley's working memory is deficient. On Digit Span, she struggled with the required cognitive manipulation of strings of numbers. It is important to note that the Digit Span subtest is more complicated than the simple, rote nature of the KABC-II NU Number Recall subtest. On Picture Span, Haley was even less able to cognitively manipulate visual

Table 1 KABC-II NU

Domain/Index and subtests	Scaled score[a]	Standard score	Percentile
Sequential processing		77	6
Number recall	9		
Word order	3		
Simultaneous processing		80	9
Rover	6		
Block counting	7		
Planning		96	39
Story completion	9		
Pattern reasoning	10		
Learning		81	10
Atlantis	7		
Rebus	6		
Knowledge		82	12
Verbal knowledge	9		
Riddles	4		
Fluid-crystallized intelligence		79	8

[a]Mean = 10; standard deviation = 3

information. The Processing Speed Domain examined the rate at which Haley could carry out mental processing. She placed consistently in the below average range in this domain.

Given Haley's Working Memory and Processing Speed rankings, her low Cognitive Proficiency standard score of 69 (2nd percentile) was to be expected. Reports of Haley's trouble with work efficiency reflect genuine, underlying weaknesses in the working memory and processing speed areas of her cognitive profile (Table 2).

Previous assessments of Haley's executive functioning were based on parent and teacher reports. Results indicated that Haley had better executive functioning in school than at home. For the current assessment, Haley's self-evaluation of her daily executive functioning was obtained using the self-report form of the Second Edition of the Behavior Rating Inventory of Executive Function (BRIEF2).

As tabulated below, Haley experiences significant struggles with executive functioning. While she is able to keep her outward behavior in check, as reflected in her acceptable Behavioral Regulation Index, her emotional regulation is more problematic: she has clinically significant difficulty when called upon to manage transitions (Shift). The cognitive regulation domain is where Haley has the most trouble, though. She acknowledged clinically significant impairments in finishing work (Task Completion) and in working memory. Overall, Haley rated her own global executive functioning with a t-score of 65 (93rd percentile), which is considered potentially clinically elevated. Haley's self-ratings, along with the findings and observations related to executive functioning discussed above, identify impaired executive functioning as a key source of some of the concerns that prompted the current assessment. Furthermore, it is important to recognize that impaired executive functioning is a common problem for individuals on the Autism Spectrum (Table 3).

Subtests on the Second Edition of the NEPSY (NEPSY-II) were utilized to examine several associated cognitive functions of Haley's. First, Haley completed the Auditory Attention and Response Set subtest to determine the extent to which distractibility could account for her struggles. She placed in the lowest percentiles on this test, indicating marked attentional difficulty both in rote attention (Auditory Attention) and in more sustained concentration (Response Set). This difficulty should be understood as a facet of Haley's Autism Spectrum Disorder.

The Comprehension of Instructions subtest required Haley to point to pictures on a card according to increasingly complex directions. Haley did well on the early,

Table 2 WISC V

Domain with subtests	Scaled score[a]	Standard score	Percentile
Working memory		65	1
Digit span	6		
Picture span	1		
Processing speed		83	13
Coding	7		
Symbol search	7		

[a]Mean = 10; standard deviation = 3

simple items but then could only do a few of the more complex items, placing in the below average range on this measure. She seemed unable to process the particular, complicated details embedded in the later instructions. Findings on this subtest confirmed that Haley has genuine trouble grasping and retaining directions.

Finally, the Narrative Memory subtest was administered. A passage was read to Haley, and she was asked a series of follow-up questions about the material covered in the passage. She answered only two questions, even with cued recall. She stated that this test was just "too hard." Again, it seemed genuinely difficult for Haley to retain much information (Table 4).

As described above, Haley completed the Beery-Buktenica Developmental Test of Visual-Motor Integration, Sixth Edition (BEERY VMI) to measure her perceptual-motor integration. Consistent with findings on other measures, Haley ranked in the below average range of visual-motor coordination, with a standard score of 83 (13th percentile). She was able to copy simple and mildly difficult shapes but could not duplicate more complex forms. At this level of ability, Haley can be expected to require effort in order to carry out graphomotor tasks at school.

It was important to gain updated information about the extent to which Haley was drawing on her abilities to learn, despite the vulnerabilities discussed up until now. For this purpose of assessing her scholastic accomplishments, selected

Table 3 BRIEF2 – Self-report form

Scale/Index	T-score[a]	Percentile
Behavioral regulation index	55	72
Inhibit	55	73
Self-monitor	54	69
Emotional regulation index	66	97
Shift	78	>99
Emotional control	53	67
Cognitive regulation index	68	95
Task completion	75	99
Working memory	72	97
Plan/organize	57	76

[a]Mean = 50; standard deviation = 10. T-scores up through 59 are acceptable. T-scores of 60-64 are mildly elevated. T-scores of 65–70 are potentially clinically elevated. T-scores of 70 and above are clinically significant

Table 4 NEPSY-II

Subtest	Scaled score[a]	Percentile
Auditory attention total		<2
Response set total		2-5
Comprehension of instructions	7	
Narrative memory	6	

[a]Mean = 10; standard deviation = 3

subtests from the Third Edition of the Kaufman Test of Educational Achievement (KTEA-3) were administered. As outlined below, at least some of Haley's academic achievement levels were remarkably good. Others were more in keeping with her intelligence scores.

In math, Haley solved word problems at a modestly average level (Math Concepts and Applications) and carried out straightforward calculations at a solidly average level (Math Computation). Even her speed was modestly average (Math Fluency).

In reading, her decoding of real words (Letter and Word Recognition) and her sounding out skills (Nonsense Word Decoding) were both modestly average. In contrast, her understanding of written material (Reading Comprehension) placed in the borderline range, as did her reading speed (Silent Reading Fluency). Thus, Haley's mechanical reading skills surpass her more conceptual, inferential skill by a significant margin. At the same time, her relatively slow mental processing interferes with reading efficiently.

In written language, the mechanics of Haley's narrative writing (Written Expression) and her spelling of isolated words (Spelling) were solidly average. However, her speed was again borderline (Writing Fluency). Also, it is very important to note that the content of her narrative writing was markedly off-topic. Asked to summarize material provided, Haley instead wrote about information that was not contained in the material. This lapse appeared related to her problems with comprehension.

In oral language, Haley was asked to listen to passages read aloud and then to answer questions about the material (Listening Comprehension). She was overwhelmed by this task and quickly reached the limit of her skills, ranking in the mildly deficient range.

Overall, it was clear that in math, mechanical areas of reading, and spelling, Haley has made excellent use of all educational efforts on her behalf and managed to meet or modestly exceed her inborn abilities. However, in reading and listening comprehension, and on tasks requiring good fluency, Haley struggles (Table 5).

Table 5 KTEA-3 – Form B

Subject	Standard score	Percentile
Math		
Math concepts and applications	91	27
Math computation	105	63
Math fluency	91	27
Reading		
Letter and word recognition	94	34
Nonsense word decoding	92	30
Reading comprehension	76	5
Silent reading fluency	76	5
Written language		
Written expression	101	53
Spelling	106	66
Writing fluency	79	8
Oral language		
Listening comprehension	68	2

As with measurements of executive functioning, previous assessments gathered information about others' views of Haley's behavioral functioning. Raters generally agreed that her behavior was usually acceptable. On the current assessment, Haley contributed her own perspective on her behavior by completing the self-report form of the Third Edition of the Behavior Assessment System for Children (BASC-3).

Haley's results on this measure are encouraging and in keeping with adult descriptions of her as pleasant and well-behaved. On the Clinical Scale, Haley was concerned only about her attentional problems; she described trouble with focusing and maintaining concentration. On the Adaptive Scale, she had concern only about her self-reliance. Item analysis indicated that Haley sees herself as a reliable and dependable person, but that she recognizes her strong need for assistance with problem-solving. Again, it is encouraging that Haley joins in the consensus that most of her behavioral functioning is appropriate, since it indicates an accurate and generally positive self-evaluation (Table 6).

The Machover Draw-A-Person Test (DAP), the Kinetic Family Drawing (KFD), and the Second Edition of the Rotter Incomplete Sentences Blank (RISB-2) were all used to gain a glimpse into Haley's internal emotional life. Results indicated that Haley believes her Autism Spectrum Disorder diagnosis is unknown to other people. Results also indicated that Haley is preoccupied with worries about the quality of

Table 6 BASC-3 – Self-report form

Scale	T-score[a]	Percentile
	Clinical	
School problems	35	4
Attitude to school	40	13
Attitude to teachers	41	22
Sensation-seeking	33	2
Internalizing problems	45	38
Atypicality	46	46
Locus of control	46	44
Social stress	41	22
Anxiety	51	61
Depression	43	25
Sense of inadequacy	47	47
Somatization	49	63
Inattention/Hyperactivity	58	78
Attention problems	66	91
Hyperactivity	48	49
Emotional symptoms	44	34
Adaptive		
Personal adjustment	50	44
Relations with parents	54	58
Interpersonal relations	55	63
Self-esteem	54	55
Self-reliance	38	13

[a]Mean = 50; standard deviation = 10. Clinical t-scores up through 59 are acceptable; of 60–69 are cause for concern; and of 70 and above are clinically significant. Adaptive t-scores of 41 and above are acceptable; of 31–40 are cause for concerns; and of 30 and below are clinically significant

her schoolwork. She is overly focused on getting good grades, with particular concern about her math progress, despite the fact that her best achievement scores are in math. Haley also evidenced an interest in rocket ships. In addition, Haley referenced the episode, discussed earlier in this report, in which she was suspended for behaving inappropriately in school. She still seemed surprised about the negative reaction to her actions. She stated that she thought that she "was just being funny" and firmly denied any bad intentions. Fortunately, other than these issues, Haley seemed relatively untroubled.

Assessment Findings Annotation

This section of the report lists and explains the results of specific test instruments. The results identify the particular aspects of Haley's capacities and skills that give rise to her difficulties regulating her behaviors and efforts. Throughout this section, evidence is being presented that will support upcoming conclusions and recommendations.

First, Haley's broad intellectual functioning is addressed, and the sufficiency of her intelligence to work productively is determined. The findings from the KABC-II NU intelligence test are presented, and the reader is guided to the correct interpretation of the scores, which is that Haley is an individual with complex, relatively weak intellectual ability.

There is a particular point to further explicate from the KABC-II NU description. In it, comments are made about the caution necessary when interpreting index and domain findings that are derived from discrepant scores. The index and domain findings are intended to describe overall, consistent abilities. If the scores that make up the index and domain findings are discrepant, then an overall finding is misrepresentative, obscuring important specific strengths and weaknesses by averaging them out. Only examining overall findings derived by discrepant scores can lead to expectations of consistent functioning that is better or worse than in reality, and thereby compromise intervention-planning. Accordingly, when significant score variability exists, it is best to examine the specific scores, rather than solely referring to overall findings.

It is often helpful to use portions of related test instruments for additional illumination of observations and issues raised by findings on core assessment measures. For Haley, a portion of a second intelligence test, the WISC V, was administered to address concerns about her cognitive efficiency. As suspected, Haley's WISC V scores documented significant working memory and processing speed problems. These problems, consistent with an Autism Spectrum Disorder diagnosis, help to explain Haley's trouble with efficient, accurate work completion.

From the WISC V description, too, there is also a particular point to further explicate. A Cognitive Proficiency score is referenced. The Cognitive Proficiency score integrates and represents abilities in working memory and processing speed.

Rather than a duplication of an overall Intelligence Quotient, the Cognitive Proficiency score is a comprehensive index of mental efficiency.

Examination of Haley's BRIEF2 protocol provides additional information about her executive functioning impairments. The footnote connected to the score table is intended to help the reader more fully understand the meaning of the scores reported. Haley's scores indicate that she experiences a good deal of difficulty with executive functioning.

It was important to finally obtain Haley's self-report of her executive functioning; doing so helped to determine if she had a reasonably accurate perspective of her own functioning. Indeed, in all psychological assessments, self-report measures provide valuable information about a youngster's self-evaluation. Comparing youth reports to caregiver and teacher reports shows the extent to which the youth is developing a view of themselves that is validated by familiar adults. In some cases, a youth's self-report indicates much more difficulty than adults' reports do. This type of discrepancy can signal that the youth is in more distress than may be outwardly evident. In other cases, a youth's self-report minimizes difficulty that is readily apparent to others. This type of discrepancy suggests significant defensiveness or distorted comprehension on the part of the youth.

Discussion of the NEPSY-II findings continues this section's effort to provide cognitive and developmental explanations for Haley's struggles with academic accuracy and efficiency. Inspection of the scores indicates that attentional problems, weakness with grasping instructions, and poor memory are all relevant to Haley's difficulties. Similarly, the BEERY VMI findings indicate that fundamental limitation in visual-motor coordination also impedes Haley's timely work completion.

The report then turns to academic achievement. Subject areas are discussed and KTEA-3 scores reported. As is done here, it is important to note and explain any contrasts between scores on different subject areas or on different components of the subject areas. Test results indicate that Haley's scholastic accomplishments are uneven but generally better than those of many of her peers on the Autism Spectrum (Schaefer Whitby & Mancil, 2009).

The next question for consideration in this report section is Haley's view of her behavioral functioning. Haley confirms the consensus that she is a generally well-behaved youngster, demonstrating accurate self-evaluation. Haley's BASC-3 scores do reveal that she is aware of experiencing moderate difficulty with distractibility and self-reliance. As with the BRIEF2 scores, the BASC-3 table's footnote helps the reader more fully understand the meaning of the specific scores reported.

This section of the report concludes with examination of the social-emotional functioning test results. Description of these results is deliberately brief, because overall findings point toward the Autism Spectrum Disorder diagnosis, rather than emotional disturbance, as a primary source of Haley's struggles. However, it is important to highlight that Haley believes her disorder is unknown to most people, despite her documented diagnostic history and evident idiosyncrasies. This inaccurate belief can be understood as consistent with the social judgment and perception difficulties that characterize individuals on the Autism Spectrum. Likewise, Haley's continued discussion of rocket ships and of the school incident indicate the perseveration that is typical of individuals on the Autism Spectrum. Additionally, while it is not surprising that Haley expresses preoccupation with her academic performance, it is interesting that she is particularly concerned about math, considering that she performs best in this subject. Her preoccupation with math in particular may be further evidence of her miscalibrated appraisals. Overall, as stated in the report, it is fortunate that Haley does not exhibit a comorbid emotional disturbance in addition to an Autism Spectrum Disorder.

Summary

Haley Smith has a long history of developmental and psychoeducational difficulties. At the time of the current assessment, she carries an Autism Spectrum Disorder diagnosis. Haley presented in a somewhat idiosyncratic manner. Still, she cooperated fully throughout the testing. Based on results from the current assessment, Haley displays below average intelligence. Supplemental testing further indicated that she has extremely low cognitive proficiency. It was apparent that Haley struggles with impaired executive functioning, attention and concentration, comprehension of instructions, and memory. Additionally, Haley's visual-motor coordination is below average. Academic achievement test results indicated a combination of solidly average and much weaker skills. Based on Haley's behavioral self-appraisal, she feels that she is doing well along most dimensions; she raised concern only about her attentional functioning and self-reliance. Findings on social-emotional tests indicated that Haley is preoccupied with rocket ships, getting good grades, and recalling an episode involving her suspension for behaving inappropriately at school.

Summary Annotation

As discussed earlier in this book, rather than presenting any new information, this section of a report should very briefly condense the findings presented in the earlier report sections. The reader should be able to obtain an accurate, concise appraisal of a youngster by reading this section of the report.

Response to Specific Referral Questions

Based on the assessment findings, it is best to offer an integrated response to the referral questions, since these questions relate to slightly different facets of the same issue. Specifically, like many individuals on the Autism Spectrum, Haley needs comprehensive external structure to do well. Appropriately, this external structure (e.g., established procedures, steady schedules, clearly prescribed expectations, role models) is much more available to her in the school setting than in the more relaxed and fluid home setting. It is clear that Haley is at a considerable disadvantage without the support of the school environment. The primary educational challenge facing Haley and her Planning and Placement Team is to determine the extent to which she can learn to generalize some of her school-based skills across settings, and then to accommodate to her limitations in attempting such generalization. A secondary challenge is to enhance Haley's overall adaptive functioning in order to improve both her educational progress and her broader quality of life.

Response to Specific Referral Questions Annotation

For assessments like Haley's that are prompted by highly specific referral questions, it is often helpful for the report to highlight direct answers to these original questions. Sometimes, as in Haley's case, the referral questions may be re-cast in light of the data obtained. To illustrate, Haley's assessment was prompted by Planning and Placement Team questions that implied that her problems were fundamentally less severe than they were, because she could perform better in school than at home. The report reorients the reader to the inborn limitations associated with Autism Spectrum Disorder, and clarifies that the reported contrast in Haley's performance between school and home environments reflects genuine deficits that are harder to manage in the latter. The report also redirects efforts on Haley's behalf by focusing on how everyone involved with her can support her across environments.

Recommendations

1. *Haley, her mother, and her educators, should take encouragement from Haley's pleasant demeanor, cooperative style, and areas of relative psychoeducational strength.*
2. *Findings from the current assessment, as well as from the Spring and Summer 2020 assessments, all support Haley's continued identification as a special education student. They also indicate that the Autism Spectrum Disorder diagnosis remains appropriate. As a special education student, Haley should continue to have year-round programming that is the most intensive possible.*
3. *Three main aspects of Haley's educational programming should be seen as critically important:*

   (a) *Executive Functioning: It is strongly recommended that Haley receive explicit instruction in executive functioning skills. In particular, she should receive assistance in monitoring her comprehension of instructions, distinguishing between required work versus non-essential tasks, identifying necessary materials for task accomplishment, and managing time.*

(b) *Social Communication: Multidisciplinary efforts should concentrate on enhancing Haley's communication with peers. Intensive effort, as well as structuring of school-based interactions, are essential to help Haley progress from limited, superficial, rote exchanges to actual verbal give-and-take.*

(c) *Social Skills: Similar multidisciplinary efforts should focus on concrete instruction and then practice in peer-to-peer social skills. While it is reassuring that Haley is rarely (if ever) negatively involved with peers, it is still very concerning that she also never actually socializes with other adolescents. Improvement of Haley's social skills is extremely important in promoting her quality of life.*

4. *Haley's educational programming should continue to provide specialized academic instruction, as needed.*

5. *In view of the fact that, at the time of the current assessment, Haley's departure from middle school is approaching, every possible effort should be aimed at achieving a smooth transition to high school. High school educators should be thoroughly informed about Haley's history and current presentation so that appropriate programming can be readied for her as a ninth grade student.*

6. *In turn, once Haley is settled comfortably into high school, it would be most important to begin to consider early transition-planning. While transition-planning typically occurs for older students, it should be expected that additional time will be needed to map out likely trajectories for Haley and then to provide suitable instruction and experiences to prepare her for appropriate future pathways.*

7. *To provide a foundation for transition-planning, Haley's high school educators should consider conducting a Futures Planning Conference. This Conference should focus on mapping out a likely young adult life for Haley and then identifying necessary skills to teach during adolescence. The document generated in the Conference could be an invaluable guide throughout Haley's high school career.*

8. *Outside of school, it is recommended strongly that parental instructional efforts focus exclusively on teaching Haley adaptive skills. Resulting improvement of Haley's adaptive behavior would be invaluable for enhancement of her self-esteem, self-reliance, and overall quality of life. Parental assistance with academic assignments should be understood as much less important for Haley's long-term success and life satisfaction.*

9. *It is recommended that Haley's mother, Ms. Smith, explore other community resources that might be helpful for Haley. Participation in adolescent recreational activities such as a gaming and movie club, martial arts instruction, swimming lessons, and therapeutic horseback riding are all examples of potentially useful and pleasant experiences for Haley.*

10. *Haley's progress should be monitored carefully. Reassessment is recommended as needed, and as required by special education regulations.*

Recommendations Annotation

As discussed earlier in this book, this section of the report begins with some opti-mism and encouragement. In the face of all the concern warranted by Haley's impairments, it is motivating to her and everyone working on her behalf to point out sources of pride and satisfaction.

The second recommendation is intended to cement the reader's understanding of Haley's diagnostic status. It should be understood fully that Haley has a lifelong developmental disorder that, by law, must be addressed vigorously.

The third recommendation directs the reader to the services that should be seen as essential to Haley's welfare. Disagreeing about home versus school performance detracts from the help that Haley requires with bolstering her executive functioning, social communication, and social skills in preparation for young adulthood.

An attempt to forestall any premature removal of special education services should be understood as the aim of the fourth recommendation.

The next few recommendations help point the way to Haley's future. Transition to adulthood is notoriously difficult for individuals on the Autism Spectrum (e.g., Anderson et al., 2018). Once the lockstep of mandatory public education is com-pleted, these individuals often flounder without the external structure on which they have relied throughout their childhood and adolescence. To help protect Haley, rec-ommendations five through seven specify approaches that could facilitate her move into a productive young adulthood.

It is important to note that a Futures Planning Conference, sometimes referred to by related names, is a gathering of everyone involved with a youngster (e.g., par-ents, caregivers, family members, educators, specialists, close friends). Whenever possible, the youngster is also involved. Through a series of specific exercises, the group takes stock of the youngster's strengths, problem areas, preferences, and needs. Participants share their hopes and dreams for the youngster, along with their concerns. Based on discussion, the group formulates a vision for the youngster's educational, vocational, and personal future. Both short- and long-term plans are made to enable the youngster to realize the vision set out by the group. A summary document is generated and can guide ongoing interventions on the young-ster's behalf.

The above recommendations focus on aspects of Haley's experience in and prog-ress through the educational system. Such a focus is appropriate, particularly given the fact that the current assessment was carried out as an independent educational evaluation requested by the Planning and Placement Team. It is also appropriate for the report to go further, though, and focus on useful goals for familial support of Haley in recommendations eight and nine. Again, Haley will benefit most from home and school ceasing to be adversarial, being as consistent as possible, and focusing on the resources and services they are best equipped to provide her.

Finally, this section concludes with a suggestion about monitoring progress and reassessing. It is necessary to remind the reader that youngsters who have been assessed almost always have difficulties that cannot be considered fully resolved directly after the assessment is completed. Reassessment is intended to follow a youngster's course and guide whatever support is necessary.

References

Anderson, K. A., Sosnowy, C., Kuo, A. A., & Shattuck, P. T. (2018). Transition of individuals with autism to adulthood: A review of qualitative studies. *Pediatrics, 141*(supplement 4), S318–S327. https://doi.org/10.1542/peds.2016-4300I

Centers for Disease Control and Prevention. (2020). *Breastfeeding facts*. https://www.cdc.gov/breastfeeding/data/facts.html

Schaefer Whitby, P. J., & Mancil, G. R. (2009). Academic achievement profiles of children with high functioning autism and asperger syndrome: A review of the literature. *Education and Training in Developmental Disabilities, 44*(4), 551–560. https://www.jstor.org/stable/24234262

Index

© Springer Nature Switzerland AG 2021

N. E. Moss, L. Moss-Racusin, *Practical Guide to Child and Adolescent Psychological Testing*, Best Practices in Child and Adolescent Behavioral Health Care, https://doi.org/10.1007/978-3-030-73515-9

Lightning Source UK Ltd.
Milton Keynes UK
UKHW020623300522
403720UK00007B/506